Titles previously published in

CANADIAN MEDICAL ASSOCIATION

This book is endorsed by the Canadian Medical Association. The association's mission is to serve and unite the physicians of Canada and be the national advocate, in partnership with the people of Canada, for the highest standards of health and health care.

Canadian Medical Association Advisors
David K. Conn MB, BCh, FRCPC
Toronto, Ontario

Duncan Robertson MB, BS, FRCP, FRCPC
Victoria, British Columbia

Jonathan P. Willmer MD, FRCPC
Ottawa, Ontario

Alzheimer's Disease

Dr. William Molloy and
Dr. Paul Caldwell

FIREFLY BOOKS

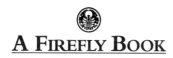

A FIREFLY BOOK

U.S. Publisher Cataloging-in-Publication Data
(Library of Congress standards)

Molloy, William.
    Alzheimer's disease: everything you need to know / William Molloy; Paul Caldwell. —1st ed.
    [224] p.: ill.; cm. (Your personal health)
Includes bibliographical references and index.
Summary: The latest developments in care, diagnosis and prognosis of those with Alzheimer's disease, with advice on how families can cope.

ISBN: 1-55297-737-4 (pbk.)

1. Alzheimer's disease – Popular works. 2. Alzheimer's disease – Social aspects. I. Caldwell, Paul. II. Title. III. Series.

616.8/ 31   21   RC523.M65 2003

Published in Canada in 2003 by Key Porter Books Limited, in conjunction with the Canadian Medical Association.

Published in the United States in 2003
by Firefly Books (U.S.) Inc.
P.O. Box 1338
Ellicott Station
Buffalo, New York, USA
14205

Diagrams: Lianne Friesen
Electronic formatting: Heidy Lawrance Associates

Printed and bound in Canada

The statements and opinions expressed herein are those of the authors, and are not intended to be used as a substitute for consultation with your physician. All matters pertaining to your health should be directed to a healthcare professional.

To my brother Frank, who has passed on. He was
the kindest soul I ever knew. God bless him and
may his soul rest in peace.

W.M.

To my father, John D. Caldwell, who always
believed in me, and to everyone who suffers,
as he did, from Alzheimer's disease.

P.C.

Contents

Acknowledgments

I would like to thank my family, Dick, Tom, John, Mary, June, Sarah and Jim, for their love, laughter, joy and support.

Thanks to my colleagues at McMaster and in Geriatric Medicine, John Kelton, Floyd Mann, Peter George, Grant Walshe, Bill Shragge, Richard Mizera, David Jewel, Kevin Sulewsky, Martin O'Donnell, Tim Standish, Christine Mitchell, Laura Jewel, Lenora Noel, Wendy McPherson, Shirley Hawkey, Rose Perovich, Karen Beretta, Chris, Judy and Garrett White, Ron and Gina Fraser, Ralph and Irmigard Schmandt, George Stallwood, Brett Sanderson, Rob Williams, Judy Lever, Rosalie Russo, Stephanie Smith, Chris Maxwell, Lee Crowe, Liza Bourcier Martin, Bill Dalziel, Kieran Sheeham, Meg Reich, Maurice and Cher Fitzgerald and Geoff Power.

D.W. M.

Much of what I have learned about the personal side of caring for Alzheimer's disease has been from the nurses and staff at the Golden Plough Lodge in Cobourg, Ontario, where my late father was a patient. Their kindness and compassion have been an inspiration to me and I am deeply grateful. I'd also like to thank Susan Delong for typing the manuscript, Dr. Chris MacKnight, Dr. Sandra Black, Dr. Allison Collins, Dr. Robert Scott, Ian and Lola Munro, and my partners, Dr. Ari Haukioja,

Dr. Michael Jones, Dr. Christine Simon and Dr. Ian Wilson. Gena K. Gorrell deserves special thanks for her wonderful direction and support as editor, as does Susan Renouf, who suggested that Dr. Molloy and I write this book together.

Writing this book has been a catharsis for me, and in trying to understand the disease I have reconciled myself to my father's fate. This process has only reinforced what I knew already—that family is everything—and I would like to thank my wife, Judy, for her support and love and my daughters Jen, Amy and Lucy for their help and encouragement. I would particularly like to thank my daughter Nina, age six, who would regularly interrupt my writing by climbing up on my lap to review the work in progress and check my spelling.

J.P.C.

Introduction

A diagnosis of Alzheimer's disease is the beginning of a long and difficult journey that lasts an average of nine years. Alzheimer's happens not only to the people who have the disease, but also to those around them. Family and friends are companions on the journey, who share the experience and the loss.

The most powerful tools to help with the disease are education, kindness and love. This book will give you the knowledge and understanding you need to let your love shine bravely and brightly all along the way.

ONE

The First Case of Alzheimer's Disease

On a cold and colorless November afternoon in 1901, a distraught husband brought his wife to the mental asylum in Frankfurt am Main for treatment. She was examined by a young German neurologist, and even at that first encounter he was perplexed by her, unable to understand or diagnose her strange symptoms and behavior. In all his medical training and experience he had never seen a case quite like this. The woman was obviously suffering from a severe alteration in her mental function, similar to what he had often seen in the very old and senile. She had the same memory loss, the same difficulty with speech, the confusion and the general feebleness of reasoning. Yet she wasn't senile. She wasn't even very old. Her problem couldn't be diagnosed as "senile dementia"—she was only 51!

Across the desk from him in the chilly examining room sat the woman, a housewife from Munich whose first name was Auguste. She appeared much older than her age. Her hair was disheveled, her clothes unkempt, and in her eyes was a wild, animal-like fear he had seen before in the mentally infirm and the truly insane. Her husband looked worn, almost haggard, but there was good reason for this. He had just finished describing his wife's unusual behavior over the last several months, and the story was heartbreaking.

She had been perfectly healthy for most of her life, had never been in the hospital, had rarely been sick. She'd worked as a laborer in a factory till they were married and children came. Now she was a *Frau* at home. She had been not only healthy but also happy, of even temper and trusting disposition—until she began to change.

He hadn't noticed it at the time but, looking back, he saw that the first hint of a problem had been her jealousy. They had enjoyed a good marriage—she had always been devoted to him. But for some reason he could not understand, she had begun to grow distrustful of him, had accused him of being unfaithful to her and angrily confronted him on several occasions. These outbursts were violent and irrational. The poor man had pleaded his innocence in front of his frightened children and professed his love, but his wife would not be satisfied. The jealousy was bad enough, but soon she began to suspect him of tricking her, and became even more agitated. He realized after a while that her memory was the problem. She would forget where she had left things—inconsequential things, such as her daughter's mittens—then fly into a rage when she couldn't locate them and accuse him of stealing and hiding them from her. These confrontations occurred frequently, with much shouting and furious agitation directed at him, for he was the object of her wrath. Such explosive fits of temper were completely out of character for his wife. Sometimes he would find things hidden in bizarre places. One time he found her hairbrush in the oven, and another time he found his pipe tucked away in the clothes for the laundry. Several times she got lost when out walking in the neighborhood. Once she went to the butcher shop half a block away, where she had shopped for years, and got quite frightened when she couldn't find her way home. He had to accompany her to be sure she was safe whenever she left to do errands.

The situation worsened. She became confused and disoriented within the confines of their small apartment—she couldn't remember where the bathroom was and she forgot the names of simple household objects such as the bed or the icebox. She could no longer cook. Not only could she not remember recipes, she couldn't remember what to do with pots and kitchen knives. She couldn't even set the table. And she had difficulty with the simplest tasks, such as dressing herself. It wasn't that she was physically incapable. Her hands and legs were still strong, and she thrashed about when she was angry—her poor husband had to hold her to stop her from beating him, so he could attest to her strength. But she had lost the will to do these simple tasks, or perhaps the understanding of the purpose behind them.

Then one night the screaming started.

Her sleep had been getting slowly worse over the months. As nighttime approached, she'd become more confused and agitated. When she finally did fall asleep (usually quite late) she often awakened later and left the bed. Her husband would follow in the dark to be sure she was safe, and watch her wander around the small apartment. Sometimes she would just stand still in the hall, or sit in a chair with a bewildered look on her face. The night she woke up screaming, she would not be soothed. The sound was unnatural, hideous. She was certain that she was about to be murdered and kept yelling, "No! No! Stop! Please!" The neighbors banged on the door to offer assistance and the husband had to assure them that his wife was simply having a bad dream.

The days that followed were agonizing. She'd pace the apartment for hours on end, sometimes dragging small pieces of furniture or bedclothes with her. Then suddenly she would pause in her wandering, cock her head as if listening and shout an answer to some voice only she heard. The couple's life was in ruins. At last the husband had brought his wife to the hospital for examination.

The portly neurologist reviewed his notes and considered the case. Although Auguste's mind was clearly gone, she had no infirmity in her body. The diagnosis wasn't insanity, nor was it any of the other mental diseases he had seen so often before. This wasn't the general paralysis of the insane seen in syphilis, or the dementia of schizophrenia. Nevertheless, it was clear that the pitiable woman in front of him had a rapidly progressive mental disease, and that she could no longer be looked after safely at home. He signed the admission papers, and she was led away into the asylum.

This encounter between the German neurologist and the *Frau* produced the first detailed description of a dementia, or loss of thinking power, that had not been recognized before, one that afflicted the middle-aged and those in their prime. We know the woman only as "Auguste D." Her personality is lost to history; her particulars, aside from the details of her illness, are forgotten. The name of the doctor, however, has become a household word. He was Dr. Alois Alzheimer.

Dr. Alzheimer

Alois Alzheimer was born in 1864 in the village of Markbreit, just outside of Würzburg in southern Germany. Following secondary school, the young Alzheimer studied medicine at the universities of Würzburg and Berlin. He graduated in 1887, after writing his final-year thesis on the functioning of the wax-producing glands of the ear. Alzheimer spent his first six months as a physician accompanying a mentally ill woman on her travels. This kind of posting was common for young physicians, and the experience gave him an interest in psychiatry and brain disorders. At the time physicians hotly debated whether the causes of mental illness were medical—that is, related to some disease of the brain or nervous tissue causing malfunction—or psychological, rooted in emotional trauma, as the influential Viennese psychiatrist Dr. Sigmund Freud claimed. Later Alzheimer obtained a job as medical officer at the mental asylum in Frankfurt am Main. By the time he met Auguste D., Alzheimer was 37 and had already established himself as a leading neurologist. He had published studies on epilepsy, brain tumors, syphilis, hardening of the arteries of the brain and other topics, and was known for his meticulous correlation of the clinical course of his patients—their complaints and his findings in hospital—with the changes that he observed after their deaths when he examined their brains under the microscope at autopsy.

Dementia

The word "dementia" comes from the Latin *de mentis*, meaning "out of the mind." The term was coined by Philippe Pinel in 1801 when he wrote about mental illness in the asylums of Paris. When used medically, the term "dementia" is very specific—it means brain failure, the inability of the brain to function normally, and it refers to a loss of intellectual ability sufficient to interfere with the person's daily activities and social or occupational life. Dementia always includes poor memory, but it also involves impaired judgment and abstract thinking, and a marked decrease in reasoning ability and insight. Dementia can be caused by such disparate things as head injuries, strokes, brain tumors and infections of the brain, but in 75 percent of those diagnosed with dementia, Alzheimer's disease is involved. The incidence of dementia rises dramatically with age, but most seniors, even those over 90, are not demented; the majority retain their faculties of reasoning, judgment and insight.

Auguste's Fate

For the next four years Auguste lived in the insane asylum in Frankfurt where Dr. Alzheimer was the admitting neurologist. They were years of anguish for both her and her family. The poor woman didn't know where she was or who she was, and after several months she failed to recognize even her husband or daughter. At first she wandered the halls of the hospital constantly, dragging sheets and bits of bedding, calling out for help. She said that she couldn't understand why she was there, that she felt confused and totally lost. She couldn't remember where her room was, nor was she able to recognize Dr. Alzheimer on his rounds. Sometimes she considered his coming an "official visit," and would apologize for not having completed her work; other times she would just scream in fear and misery. On several occasions Auguste sent the

---

Senility

The word "senility" comes from the Latin *senium*, meaning "old"; the adjective "senile" (old) simply means the opposite of "juvenile" (young). The term has nothing to do with mental function or ability; it refers to age alone. In Alzheimer's time, it was believed that most if not all persons would lose their mental faculties as they aged—that is, they would become demented—and the term "senile" became associated with this loss. We now know that this is not the case. Age does not necessarily bring about significant decreases in reasoning powers or mental abilities. In fact, age can allow a wealth of experience and the altered perspective we call wisdom. Auguste D. developed dementia at a very early age— before senility (old age)—and for years her condition was labeled "pre-senile" dementia. We now know that the Alzheimer's disease that occurs at a young age is the same disease that occurs in older people. We also know that although Alzheimer's disease becomes more common with age, it is certainly not inevitable. Thomas Jefferson founded the University of Virginia at age 65; Goethe finished *Faust* in his middle seventies; George Bernard Shaw began writing his first novel after the age of 60 and Verdi was 79 when he composed the great opera *Falstaff*. So much for senility!

doctor away with a string of curses, telling everyone in attendance that he was making sexual advances toward her. She had a curious way of talking and would mix up words, often not using the precise word needed but rather words of similar or related meaning—she would say "milk jug," for example, instead of "cup." Many nights she screamed for hours, a horrible, inhuman wail that echoed up and down the dark stone corridors of the asylum.

Auguste worsened year by year. Eventually she became bedridden, forced by contractures to lie on her side like an infant, her legs drawn up and her arms curled across her chest. She had large, fetid bedsores and was incontinent, and she was completely unaware of her surroundings. Four and a half years after her disease had first shown itself as jealousy toward her husband, Auguste D. died at the age of 55, undiagnosed and alone, a frail shell of the woman she had once been.

The Signs in Auguste's Brain

For four years, as he watched her decline in the asylum, Dr. Alzheimer was puzzled by the strange mental disease of Auguste D. But it was only several days after she died—after her brain was removed from her skull and stained so that various cell types could be identified—that the neurologist was able to investigate the disease that had so ravaged his patient.

He began by studying her brain as a unit. After weighing it, he held it gently in his hands and turned it round and round, inspecting its minute details. It was certainly smaller than it should have been, perhaps by a third, and lighter than expected, and it appeared shriveled. Normally, the outer layer of the human brain is so massive and well developed that it must fold back on itself to fit inside the skull. The resulting accordion-like pleats of this outer layer of brain are known as the cerebral cortex (*cortex* from the Latin for "tree bark"; the human cortex looks like wet bark). Alzheimer noticed immediately that these pleats were much thinner than usual in Auguste D., with wide areas between them—as if the very tissue of the brain had wasted away.

Next, Alzheimer looked through his microscope at thinly sliced pieces of brain tissue. As a result of advances in staining techniques and German optics technology, he had become one of the leading European specialists in diseases of the brain, particularly the microscopic changes evident in the various disorders that cause neurological signs. What he saw in the brain of Auguste D. were the characteristics of a new dementia.

The first thing Alzheimer noted was that many of the expected brain cells were not visible—they were simply not there. He could see the empty sites where they had once been, but the neurons (the basic cells of the brain responsible for all neurological thinking and activity) had disappeared.

Brain Cells Choked by Strange Tangled Fibers

Many of the remaining neurons were definitely not normal—in their cell bodies they had strange, threadlike, spindle-shaped objects that were very prominent and absorbed the stain well, becoming dark under the microscope. Some cells had only one or two of these unusual filaments, but in other cells the fibers were matted side by side in bundles so thick that they appeared to be choking the neurons. In the worst cases, the neurons had all but disappeared, leaving only a tangled mass of coarse, ropelike structures. Alzheimer called these filaments "fibrils"— meaning small fibers—and the presence of groups of these fibers in layers throughout the cerebral cortex is a diagnostic microscopic sign of Alzheimer's disease.

These "neurofibrillary tangles" (as Alzheimer labeled them) appeared in many cells in Auguste's brain—he estimated between one-quarter and one-third of the brain had the dark, threadlike rods that filled up and overpowered the normal cells. No wonder the poor woman couldn't reason properly! Alzheimer postulated that since the fibrils had stained differently from normal brain tissue, and since they had survived the destruction of the cell, they must have undergone some sort of chemical transformation. He wrote: "It seems that the transformation of these fibrils goes hand in hand with the storage of an as yet not closely examined disease-producing product of metabolism in the neuron." Time has shown the careful German neurologist to be right. Understanding the cause of the twisted fibers he observed is crucial to understanding the disease process.

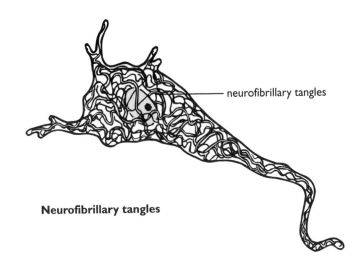

neurofibrillary tangles

Neurofibrillary tangles

Plaquelike Scars in the Brain

There were other unusual microscopic findings. Dispersed over the entire surface of the brain, the barklike cortex, were large numbers of thick, viscous-looking blobs that Alzheimer called "plaques." Through the microscope it looked as if someone had splattered globs of paint across the cortex. These plaques were so prominent that they could be recognized even on a cut section of the brain that had not been stained, as a large number of dense, irregularly edged black spots—very foreign-looking, like microscopic craters in a biological battlefield. The unusual plaques had been identified before, in the brains of the very old—Alzheimer recognized them as the so-called senile plaques. These three pathological changes in the brain— the loss of brain cells, the mats of destructive fibers he called "neurofibrillary tangles" and the senile plaques—were Alzheimer's chief findings after he examined Auguste's brain. A century later, they remain the basis for the microscopic diagnosis of the disease.

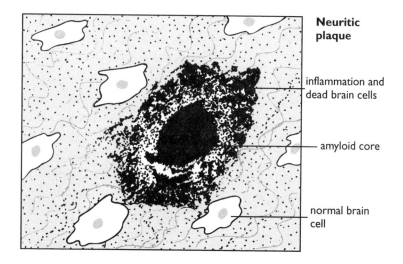

Neuritic plaque

inflammation and dead brain cells

amyloid core

normal brain cell

Several months after the autopsy on Auguste was concluded, Alzheimer presented the case to a group of psychiatrists at a meeting in southern Germany in 1906—with the first published description of this new dementia. He stressed the clinical deterioration in one so young, the shrunken brain and the presence of so many senile plaques along with the strange tangles of fibrils. He concluded that "It is evident that we are dealing with a peculiar little-known disease process." How prophetic his conclusion was!

Alzheimer's Later Years

At the time he presented the strange case of Auguste D., Dr. Alzheimer was at Heidelberg University, where he taught neurology and histology, the newly founded science of examining diseased tissue microscopically. He was a revered teacher and students came from all around the world to his laboratory. He smoked constantly and used to set down his lit cigar beside a student's instrument in order to demonstrate the significant points of the microscopic examination. So enthusiastic and absorbed was he that by the end of the day half-smoked cigars sat beside every microscope. Others began to refer to the case not as that of Auguste D., but as the disease Dr. Alzheimer had observed. (The habit of naming a disease after the physician who first described it was well established at the time—Parkinson's disease and Huntington's chorea are well-known examples.) Soon other neurologists began to recognize similar cases, and confirmed Alzheimer's microscopic findings as being diagnostic.

In 1912, Alzheimer accepted a position as full professor at University Hospital in the German town of Breslau. As he was traveling by train to his new appointment, he fell ill with acute streptococcal tonsillitis—"strep throat." Before the age of antibiotics, tonsillitis was a serious infection, and he spent several weeks in the hospital. He was left with heart damage from rheumatic fever, a complication of his tonsillitis, and spent the next three years in the hospital with increasing weakness and heart disease. He died in 1915 of endocarditis, a form of heart valve infection, and kidney failure. He was 51 years old—the same age as Auguste D. when she first came to him with the strange disease that now bears his name.

How Common Is Alzheimer's Disease?

"The disease of the century" is what the scientist Lewis Thomas called Alzheimer's, and there is good evidence to support his claim. Fear of "losing one's mind" is the greatest single worry of our aging population; this dread of loss of mental faculties, and thus of personal control, is greater than the fear of cancer, heart disease, arthritis or other painful conditions, or indeed any other aspect of aging. Unfortunately, for many seniors this fear becomes a terrifying reality.

The incidence of Alzheimer's—and other dementias—is directly related to age. Though some verified cases have been diagnosed in people still in their twenties, these are exceedingly rare, as is the diagnosis before the age of 50. From studies done around the world we know that dementia occurs in approximately 8 percent of all people over 65, though the incidence varies from country to country and study to study. It occurs in approximately 25 percent of those over 80, and up to 40 percent of those over 90. This means that almost one in ten of the population we consider "seniors" has dementia of some kind. It also means that of those who survive to age 90 or greater, about one in three will be demented.

These days our population is aging and our life expectancy is increasing. Five hundred years ago it was unusual to be aged; people died younger. Over the past several centuries, improvements in nutrition, public health measures to prevent disease and illness and advances in medicine have protected us from premature death, so that a larger and larger percentage of our population lives decades longer. Because we are living longer, degenerative brain diseases such as Alzheimer's now pose a major health problem to our society. With further improvements in medical care, we expect that a larger percentage of our population will be able to live comfortably into their eighties and nineties—and this means that the incidence of

Alzheimer's around the world

Alzheimer's may be four times more common in British men than in North American and Japanese men. British women may be three times more likely to get Alzheimer's than Japanese women are. It's not clear why there is such variation. It may be genetics, diet, the environment or other unknown factors. Or it may simply be that the disease is diagnosed and reported differently in these countries.

Cases of Alzheimer's disease per 100,000 population

	Men	Women
Japan	.8	1.5
Russia	1.1	3.8
Scandinavia	1.6	2.2
Britain	3.0	4.9
U.S.A./Canada	.7	2.1

Alzheimer's disease will rise dramatically over the next few decades. Half the children born in Canada this year are expected to live 81 years or more, and approximately one in four will develop a severe dementia such as Alzheimer's. Alzheimer's disease has become the fourth-leading cause of death in the United States, and one family in three has a member with a dementia problem. By enabling our citizens to grow older, we have changed the pattern of disease and death in our society.

Alzheimer's in Canada

To understand the scope of these changes, consider the figures for the aged population in Canada. In 1900, 5 percent of Canadians were over 65. The figure rose to 10 percent in 1991. It was predicted to reach 12 percent by the year 2000, and it is projected that by 2031 fully 21 percent of Canadians will be over 65. This means that over only a century and a third the percentage of Canadians over 65 will have more than quadrupled—an incredible increase.

Alzheimer's disease is reported to be by far the commonest type of dementia. A 1994 study estimated that by 2002 more than 300,000 Canadians would suffer from Alzheimer's. There are 10,000 new cases diagnosed each year—27 cases a day. Twice as many females as males are diagnosed as having dementia in Canada and, as elsewhere in the world, the prevalence of dementia of any kind is very much age related. In Canada only 2.4 percent of those aged 65 to 74 are demented, but this figure rises to 34.5 percent in those 85 or older. As the Canadian population ages, the incidence of dementia is predicted to increase dramatically. According to the same study, by the year 2030 three-quarters of a million cases of dementia are expected in Canada—an increase of 300 percent over present figures; the population will have increased by only 40 percent.

The cost of caring for dementia is incredibly high—higher than the cost of caring for stroke and cancer combined. In Canada this cost was estimated in 1991 at $3.9 billion— 6 percent of the nation's total health costs for that year. The 1994 study estimated that by the year 2030 the cost would rise to $12 billion a year. (A new study is expected in the near future.)

Alzheimer's in the U.S.A.

The situation is similar in the United States. It is estimated that in 2000 Alzheimer's disease affected four million Americans and that it kills 100,000 each year, and these figures will become even more alarming as the nation ages. In 1900 there were three million seniors (over age 65) in America, and in 1980 there were 25 million—an eightfold increase. It's estimated that there were about 31 million people over the age of 65 in the year 2000. The figures are even more startling for the "very old," those over 75. In 1900 there were only 900,000 "very old" in the U.S., but by 1980 there were 10 million.

(There are presently over 50,000 seniors in the U.S. who are over 100 years old.) According to estimates, in the year 2000 there were more than 13 million persons over age 75 living in the U.S., and approximately one in four of them was demented. The cost of caring for those with Alzheimer's disease in the United States in 1992 was estimated at $100 billion a year—a figure that is almost unimaginable.

Alzheimer's As a Global Problem

By the year 2020 there will likely be a billion people on this planet who are over age 60, and it seems clear that as the population ages, the incidence of Alzheimer's disease (and other dementias) will rise proportionately. Each of the individuals with Alzheimer's will survive an average of nine years, and most will require ongoing care either at home or in the hospital for the duration of their illness. They will have a progressive decline in mental function to the point where they are no longer able to look after themselves and are completely dependent on others for their safety, personal hygiene, nutrition and medical care. This will place an incredible burden on the health care systems of our countries, as well as be an overwhelming practical and emotional responsibility for our citizens and families.

Close-up of a Brain

Alzheimer's disease is an affliction of the brain. It is the brain alone that is "diseased." All the signs and symptoms of Alzheimer's—from the earliest difficulties with memory to the last stages before death—are the result of damage to cells within the brain; the disease impairs the function of these cells at a microscopic level, causing the deterioration in mental ability and behavior that we observe on a day-to-day basis.

To understand what areas of the brain are involved in the disease, and how damaged brain cells in these areas produce symptoms, let's take a brief look at the anatomy and function of a normal brain, then see what happens in the Alzheimer's brain.

The Cortex

If you look inside the skull to examine the human brain, the first anatomical structure you come across is a shining clear membrane called the *dura mater*, the outer layer of the *meninges*, membranes that hold many of the brain's important blood vessels and envelop the brain like tough plastic wrap. Below this protective cover is the brain itself. The wrinkled exterior, the *cortex*, is packed with millions of neurons. These working cells of the brain—what we think of as "brain cells"—are a light gray in color. The processes that lead away from the neurons (and that carry impulses away from the cell bodies) are a whitish color. Thus, "gray matter" refers to the actual bodies of the brain cells, while "white matter" refers to the elements that carry impulses away from these cell bodies.

Brain areas

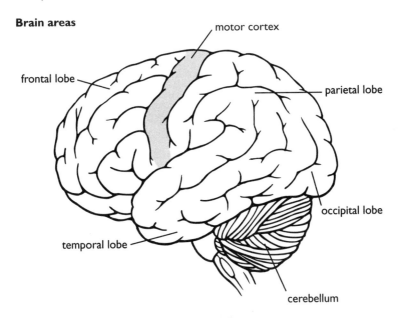

It is the cortex that makes us human, for within this thin exterior layer of the brain lies our ability to plan, calculate, imagine and create. But there is something more. We know that when the cortex of the brain functions normally, it creates a person, someone with a particular pattern of feelings, beliefs, reactions and thoughts, and these transcend the purely physical. A working cortex produces an individual pattern of emotion, aspiration and experience that defines the character and the personality.

Unfortunately, it is the cortex, this brain-cell layer half an inch (1.25 cm) thick on the surface of the brain, that is most affected by Alzheimer's disease.

The Divisions of the Cortex

The cortex is divided into four kinds of large areas, or lobes, each responsible for particular functions. The largest is the *frontal lobe*, and it takes up the front one-third of the brain, directly above the face. The frontal lobe is responsible for insight, planning and organization. It's also responsible for personality and initiative. There are two *temporal lobes*, one at each temple. These are very important in Alzheimer's disease because this is where the function of memory resides. Other temporal lobe functions include the processing and interpretation of sounds and the formation and understanding of speech. The *parietal lobes* ("parietal" means "wall" or "side") are located on the crown of the brain, at the top and at the back. These areas of cortex integrate the input from the senses of vision, touch and hearing. The parietal lobes are also responsible for the recognition and use of numbers. The *occipital lobe* is at the back of the skull, just above the neck, and it is responsible for the processes of vision.

At the center of the brain, just above where the spinal cord begins, is another large collection of neurons. They are responsible for more basic functions, such things as thirst and hunger, sexual drive, the regulation of temperature and the level of alertness. This area is called the *midbrain*. Attached on its back, or posterior, side is a wrinkled swelling called the *cerebellum*. It is responsible for the complicated processes of movement. It is affected in Alzheimer's disease only late in the course of the illness.

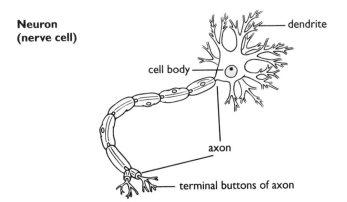

**Neuron
(nerve cell)**

cell body

dendrite

axon

terminal buttons of axon

Association Pathways and Areas

Each specialized area of the cortex is connected to all the other areas by specific *association pathways* that quickly transmit information from one area to another to integrate information from multiple sites. Interconnectedness occurs throughout the brain; one area of the brain always knows what the other areas are doing—are "thinking." The association pathways must function well in order for the different areas of the brain to work together. In addition to the pathways, there are specific areas of the brain in which input from several other areas is summarized and coordinated. These are called *association areas*, for they associate (or combine) the information from several different areas into one congruent picture. For example, while you are reading this book, the individual letters on the page are being "associated" into meaningful words by your temporal and occipital lobes, and (we hope) your frontal lobe is giving you new insight into the complex functioning of the brain. All this is happening without your being aware of it—and you take the process for granted—but in Alzheimer's disease, damage to the association pathways and association areas is dramatic and severe. Many of the clinical signs and symptoms of the disease result from destruction of these key areas within the brain. This damage causes the various areas of the brain to become isolated, to work alone, without input from other areas of the brain, so that no "total picture" is formed. Thus, someone with Alzheimer's disease may be able to read the words in this sentence, but not be able to connect them to form an idea and derive any meaning from them.

Brain Cells

Though the human brain is an incredible piece of biology, its microscopic anatomy is fairly simple and easily understood. Under magnification, brain tissue is seen to be composed of only two types of specialized cells: neurons and *neuroglia*.

The word "neuron" comes from the Greek, meaning "nerve," and neurons are responsible for all the mental processes that go on in the brain. These "thinking" cells of the brain die in large number in Alzheimer's disease.

The other cells in the brain, called *neuroglia* (from the Greek for "nerve," plus *glia*, meaning "glue"), form supporting tissue for the neurons. They also provide the neurons with essential nutrients, help the neurons to conduct impulses, and repair nerve-cell damage. Thus, they are essential to proper neuron (and brain) function. These cells become inflamed in Alzheimer's disease.

Each neuron has a cell wall and nucleus, just like many other cells in the body. Each neuron also has numerous tiny finger-like projections from the cell body, called *dendrites* (from the Greek for "tree"). These dendrites branch out from the main part of the cell just as branches do from the trunk of a tree.

Because these dendrites are essential to the proper function of a brain cell, there are large numbers of them per neuron—anywhere from several hundred up to 200,000. Each of the hundreds or thousands of dendrites on each neuron is in contact with at least several dendrites from other neurons in the vicinity. Some connect with up to 15,000 others! Imagine a whole forest of trees jammed together right side up, upside down, sideways, so that their branches and leaves intertwine. This is what the brain looks like microscopically. This huge mass of interlocking dendrites allows a single neuron to communicate with many, many other neurons—a very important task of brain tissue that allows coordination of brain function.

Dendrites bring information to a neuron. *Axons*, on the other hand, take information away from a neuron. In contrast to its many dendrites, each neuron has only one axon, but at its end the axon branches out into many smaller fingerlike processes to touch other cells. An important component of the axon is the system of hollow cylinders called *microtubules*. These convey electrical and chemical impulses quickly along the axon's length. They are severely damaged in Alzheimer's disease, becoming twisted into the neurofibrillary tangles seen throughout the brain.

Neuron Meets Neuron: The Synapse

Neurons don't exactly touch each other. They are separated by a very tiny space—the *synapse*. The space is not empty, but filled with a rich and complex soup of brain chemicals. Messages are passed from one neuron to another across this tiny gap. It is worth understanding this process, as many of the drugs used to treat Alzheimer's disease have their effects on these chemicals. When a neuron sends a message—actually a combination of electrical and chemical information—to another neuron, the message travels from the cell body down the axon to the fine, fingerlike projections at its very end. There it causes specific changes in the chemical soup between the neurons. Brain chemicals called *neurotransmitters* (literally, brain-cell transmission agents) cross the gap between axon and dendrite. They are released at the axon, then picked up at the dendrite. In this way the message or information is passed across.

Synapse

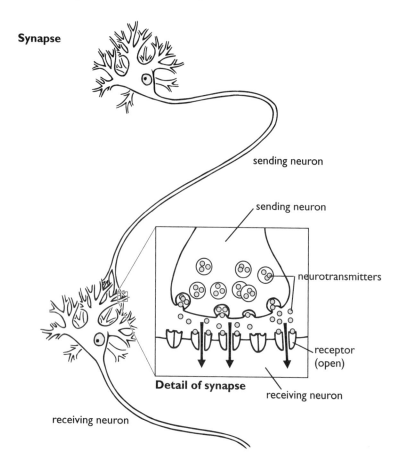

sending neuron

sending neuron

neurotransmitters

receptor (open)

Detail of synapse

receiving neuron

receiving neuron

Neurotransmitters are markedly reduced in Alzheimer's disease, particularly the neurotransmitter *acetylcholine*. This means that the messages cannot get across the gap between neurons, or do so only slowly or incompletely. The wonderful system of communication between brain cells, the synapse, has been dramatically altered by the disease.

What Is Wrong with the Alzheimer's Brain?

People with Alzheimer's disease demonstrate progressive signs of mental impairment because of microscopic damage to individual neurons in the brain. This damage does not occur uniformly throughout the brain; it is much more severe in some areas than in others, and always begins in specific regions. If you examined the brain early in the disease you'd see a "motheaten" effect in certain places only. The functions that correspond to these anatomical places would be markedly reduced or abnormal. However, right beside this damaged anatomical area, other brain cells might very well be functioning fairly normally. As the disease progresses, more and more tissue within the brain is damaged, and a progressive general decline in mental ability is the result. At death, most of the brain is involved, although even then some areas are much more damaged than others.

There are many microscopic changes that occur in Alzheimer's disease, but the most important ones are the three that Alzheimer noted in the brain of Auguste D.—neuron loss, the formation of senile (also called *neuritic*) plaques and the

---

Alzheimer's and education

Education defends against Alzheimer's; people who have received more education seem to be resistant to the disease. This finding could have a number of explanations. People with a lot of education may live in a higher socioeconomic bracket and their lifestyle may protect them. For example, people who have less education may work in more manual jobs with more exposure to head injuries and environmental toxins, and may have poorer diets and receive less health care. Repeated brain activity may somehow protect the brain from decay. Some people may simply have more complex brains than others, and thus have more reserves and tolerate damage better. Another possible explanation is that people with Alzheimer's had poor memories as early as childhood and did not receive more education because this problem affected their ability to learn.

accumulation of neurofibrillary tangles—as well as the marked destruction of the synapses and the loss of neurotransmitters. These microscopic changes cause the signs and symptoms of the disease.

Is Alzheimer's accelerated brain aging?

None of the pathological microscopic changes in the brain—the loss of neurons, the senile plaques, the neurofibrillary tangles—is specific to Alzheimer's disease, or by itself diagnostic of it. Normal aging produces some thinning of the cortex (because of neuron loss) and often a few scattered plaques, as well. Even neurofibrillary tangles occur in the aged brain, in perfectly normal individuals. The difference is that in Alzheimer's disease these changes occur in much greater numbers. Because these changes are seen in normal aging (although to a very much reduced degree), it may be that all of us have some of the processes that produce these cell changes operating in our brains—that is, all of us may have some degree, though minimal, of the damage from Alzheimer's disease as we age. Conversely, some have argued that because some degree of senile plaques and neurofibrillary tangles is seen in normal aging, Alzheimer's may be viewed as an accelerated aging of the brain.

THREE

Finding the Pattern: Common Signs and Symptoms

For most families, the disturbing progression of mental and physical changes that Alzheimer's disease brings to their loved one produces a sense of loss that is monumental. Day after day the person they once knew and loved changes, often in bizarre ways, until one day only faint traces of the former person remain. Their husband or father, their wife or daughter, has been replaced by a bewildered stranger.

As difficult as it is to lose a loved one, with Alzheimer's disease the loved one is not only lost but to some extent replaced—the disease seems to take over the mind, and thus the personality and the character, leading to an endless series of confrontations, disputes and failures, a collection of seemingly haphazard and often grotesque symptoms of mental decline. Though relentless in its destruction, this decline appears completely unpredictable to the family, who are overwhelmed not only by the disease but by its apparently aimless and indiscriminate destruction.

However, studies of thousands of people with the disease have shown what patterns of behavior and mental decline tend to occur, and which are most common. We know that the changes are a direct result of individual brain cells being damaged by the pathological processes of Alzheimer's disease. We also know that, at least initially, not all cells in the brain are damaged equally. Some seem much more susceptible, and are destroyed much earlier in the course of the disease. By referring to these studies, we are much better able to predict the symptoms and changes in behavior, and even to understand them.

Almost all cases of Alzheimer's begin with the same complaints, progress through the same gradual decline and end up in the same terminal phase. Of course, every individual is different, and no two cases are exactly alike—but many prob-

Dignity and Alzheimer's disease

The concept of dignity is a very important one in understanding Alzheimer's, particularly in maintaining respect for someone who has the disease. Just as the smoothly functioning collection of neurons we call the normal brain creates a mind and produces a personality, so damage to these cells produces changes in the mind and personality. The confusion, the memory loss, the agitation, even the striking out at loved ones and the eventual loss of recognition of spouses and children are a direct result of damage to specific cells within the brain, just as the pain of a heart attack is the direct result of damage to heart muscle. Because the brain is so much more complex in its normal function than the heart, it becomes more grotesque in dysfunction. Through no fault of their own, Alzheimer's sufferers change in mind and personality because of microscopic damage to the brain that accumulates as time passes. As the disease progresses and more and more brain cells become damaged, moods, attitudes, memories and other facets of personality deteriorate inexorably. Eventually the person we used to know vanishes. By recognizing that this is the direct result of *physical damage*, we can respect people with Alzheimer's, preserve their dignity and appreciate them for who they were before the disease attacked them.

lems are shared by most people with the disease. A working knowledge of the usual course of Alzheimer's allows some comfort for both the person who has the disease and the family, as the changes become less unexpected and confusing. This chapter explores the common signs and symptoms of Alzheimer's. (Signs are effects the doctor can observe, like impaired speech; symptoms are effects that have to be noted by the patient, such as headache.)

Memory Changes
Usually the first problem recognized is a disturbance of the complicated phenomenon we call "memory."

In the first year or so of his retirement, John and his wife, Sally, had a wonderful time. John had worked as a machine operator in a plastics plant, and because of his organizational and people skills he had been promoted to the personnel department for his last years with the company. He had always had a good memory and he prided himself on knowing everyone in the plant. An avid fisherman and outdoorsman, he spent his winter evenings tying trout flies or planning fishing trips. Summers were filled with adventurous fishing, camping and other outdoor activities.

But after a while he realized that something was wrong. He just couldn't seem to trust his mind the way he once had—particularly his memory. It wasn't that he couldn't remember at all—he could still reel off the names of members of his high-school football team, or the specific formula for calibrating the extruding machine he had used for eight years at the plant. It was more that he couldn't *count* on his memory. Simple things, such as the date of his granddaughter's birthday or the exact weekend the fishing season opened—these things he couldn't remember, no matter how hard he tried. He'd gotten a new license plate the year before, but the numbers still wouldn't come to him when he paid for gas at the service station. He had to print the numbers on a small piece of paper and keep it folded in the glove compartment. His son and daughter-in-law had recently moved, and John loved talking to them and his four-year-old granddaughter on the phone, but he couldn't for the life of him remember their new phone number, though the old one came to him with ease. Lately he was convinced that his mind was failing—not just playing tricks on him, but not functioning well.

One day John went to the corner store to pick up a few things, but when he entered the store he had absolutely no idea why he had come. Sheepishly he bought a package of gum and a newspaper, and then, shaken by the incident, he sat in his car outside, trying to make sense of what had happened. Sally constantly told him he was repeating himself, telling the same stories, asking the same questions again and again, and several times, after they had casually run into friends when they were out walking, he'd had to ask her their names, even though he knew he had grown up with them. Understandably, he was becoming unsure of himself, and withdrawing from much of his social contact. He didn't want to be humiliated. He allowed his wife to do more and more for him. He had always carefully reviewed the bank statements each month, but now he seemed uninterested in them and she had to look after them. One evening when they were watching television, he casually asked her what they were going to have for supper—only to be told that they had eaten less than an hour before.

The worst episode was at Christmastime. John was devoted to Sally, and he bought her a beautiful, expensive silver locket and necklace, a reflection of his love for her. On Christmas morning he was very excited about giving it to her, and he hurried through the other presents in anticipation. Unfortunately, he couldn't find it. He had hidden it away several days

Common signs and symptoms of Alzheimer's disease

- loss of memory, especially recent memories
- inability to learn, to process new information
- language difficulties
- poor judgment and reasoning ability, leading to self-neglect and carelessness
- spatial disorientation: getting lost, avoiding trips
- behavioral changes: sleep disorders, hallucinations and delusions, disturbances in activity levels, aggression and mood disturbances

before Christmas, and now he couldn't remember where it was. He was embarrassed and ashamed, and then panic-stricken. It was awful, the two of them searching the house together for this symbol of his love, while he felt more and more desperate and she felt more and more empty. He did find the locket, quite by accident, two days after Christmas, but by that time his joy in giving such a present had been replaced by a hollow sadness.

What Memory Means to Us

Our sense of identity—who we are—depends to a large degree on our ability to remember. We are all defined by our own specific collections of personal and distinctive experiences, encounters and achievements. These characterize us, delineate us, and all depend on our ability to recall the past at will. Our occupations, hobbies, interests, our learning and our relationships with others (even those we love), build layer on layer on what has gone before. Being unable to remember is a threat to our very being as thinking creatures.

Imagine what the world would be like if you couldn't trust your memory—if you couldn't recall the details of your life. How upset would you feel if you couldn't remember the names of your nearest and dearest or the particulars of your job—or even such simple things as what you had for breakfast? You would be trapped forever in the present, without any recourse to the past for understanding or comfort. Experience would be worthless to you; every second would be a new beginning, everywhere you looked a new exploration, every encounter a new introduction. We all feel anxious with any change—it's a normal human trait—and we feel most secure in environments and circumstances that we've had previous experience with—that is, that we've learned are safe. Imagine the constant state of agitation, of stress, if you couldn't trust your memory. You would be permanently lost: unable to orient yourself from moment to moment or to familiarize yourself with a new scene or situation. You might feel that you had to go to the bathroom, yet be unable to remember where the bathroom was. You might meet the same "new people" again and again, all day long. You might not be certain what you had had for lunch (or even whether you'd eaten), or what you had done the day before. A thousand scraps of knowledge might elude you—where you had put your bedroom slippers, whether today was the day your daughter was coming over, if you had turned off the burner under the coffeepot. Stripped of the stability and reassurance that memory provides, you would be in a state of constant apprehension.

Most studies of Alzheimer's disease indicate that forgetfulness or memory loss is the very first sign that something is truly wrong; memory loss is the single most common reason people seek medical aid. Moreover, a significant loss of the ability to remember is an essential factor in the diagnosis, so much so that the disease cannot be diagnosed unless it is present. You simply cannot have Alzheimer's disease and at the same time have normal memory.

To understand how memory is damaged by Alzheimer's disease, you first need an understanding of the complicated process of normal memory.

The Nature of Memories

The word "memory" refers specifically to the ability to retain or recall thoughts, images, ideas, experiences and whatever you have previously learned. Though all animals, even very simple ones, have "memory" (even an amoeba can be taught to avoid a noxious stimulus), the ability to store information and later retrieve it is one of the most important achievements of human intelligence. Our ability to remember is responsible for much of our success as a species, for memory allows us to learn as a community, to profit from previously acquired information even if we did not acquire it personally. Memory and learning are seamlessly intertwined, and though we take them for granted, these two very human skills are responsible for all of our reasoning, calculating and planning, and most of our everyday thinking.

Throughout our lives we are constantly bombarded with information. Memory is our way of processing this information as it is presented to us, sorting out what is useful from what is not and recording for future use whatever our minds select as significant. Without an adequately functioning memory we become lost, childlike, unable to process any new information in a meaningful way.

The phenomenon of human memory can be divided into three interrelated stages—immediate, short-term and long-term. Though the effects of Alzheimer's disease on memory are marked, not all aspects of memory are equally damaged. A working knowledge of how the disease affects each of these stages allows us to understand many of the changes that occur early in the disease.

Immediate Memory

The term "immediate memory" refers to information that has just been presented to us. For example, the words you are now reading in this sentence form an immediate memory, as does your awareness of the temperature of the room you are in, the quality of the light you are reading by and so on. If you were given a short list of unrelated words and then asked to repeat the list, it would be a test of your immediate memory. Another term used by psychologists for this ability is "working memory," signifying that this kind of memory allows you to manipulate information rapidly in your mind without necessarily retaining it. Doing simple arithmetic is a good example of this kind of memory in action. Only the final number, the answer, is important, so the various numbers calculated in the process of the arithmetic are noted in immediate, or working, memory but quickly forgotten. Immediate memory holds information that is not meant to be remembered for long. It's like a blackboard in a schoolroom: information is noted on it, but the entries will soon be erased, except when the mind decides that something is worth saving and elects to process it into the next stage, short-term memory.

Immediate memory is well preserved until the later stages of Alzheimer's disease.

Short-term Memory

If your mind decides that something is worth remembering, the information proceeds to another anatomical site in your brain, where it can be stored and kept available for rapid retrieval. This is short-term memory. However, short-term memory has a very limited capacity—you can't hold a lot of information here. Information in short-term memory is not completely "learned" (that is, able to be retrieved forever). Short-term memory is a holding bank, a limited container for information that will be retained for a relatively brief period of time. For example, you are given a telephone number to call in a little while and you know it's important to remember it. Your immediate recall of the telephone number (simply repeating the number) does not ensure that you will be able to remember it in two or three hours, when you need it. Thus, you must transfer the information from immediate memory into short-term memory, a process called "encoding." In order to accomplish this you must reinforce the memory in your mind. With telephone numbers you do so by repeating the number again and again, until your mind forms a sequence that allows you to recall it at will.

Because the short-term memory system has limited capacity, it is difficult to commit to memory more than a few pieces of information at once—one telephone number, for instance. The average adult can easily remember seven or eight unrelated numbers, but most adults cannot remember more than ten or eleven in a row. When the capacity of short-term memory is full, you are aware that you can't remember anything more.

The information held in short-term memory will fade with time unless it's rehearsed again and again or is deemed significant enough to proceed to the last stage of memory, long-term memory.

Short-term memory is a pivotal element in the processing of newly acquired information—identifying what is important enough to be remembered and what is not. A properly functioning short-term memory system allows important information to be transferred from immediate recall to long-term memory. It is impossible to learn without this facility; such simple tasks as orienting yourself in a new room or building, recalling a short shopping list, keeping a bridge score or remembering errands all become impossible when short-term memory fails.

Short-term memory is usually severely affected early in the course of Alzheimer's disease. In fact, much of the difficulty with remembering that is so often the first sign of Alzheimer's occurs in this critical stage of memory processing.

Long-term Memory

This is what we think of as true memory: information that can be recalled at will over an extended period of time, often a lifetime. Examples include the names of your cousins or fellow employees, a family recipe, your anniversary date and many of the pieces of information important to occupations. This kind of information has been consolidated into a comprehensive unit, available for recall and examination in a complete form at virtually any time. This is also the area of memory that makes us wise. As we age, the amount of information we hold, what we "know," increases tremendously, and our ever-growing accumulation of experiences, encounters and knowledge gives us a perspective we didn't have when we were younger.

Because it is held in a different anatomical site in the brain from short-term memory, long-term memory is often surprisingly little affected until late in Alzheimer's disease.

The "Information Secretary"

Information often shifts through the three stages of memory without our being aware of it—we take the process for granted—but the mechanism of memory may be clearer if we compare the process to the filing of documents in an office. To begin with, some sort of information is deemed to be important and the secretary types the information, as individual words, onto sheets of paper; this process is equivalent to the formation of an immediate, or working, memory. Next, the secretary may choose to gather several sheets of that typed

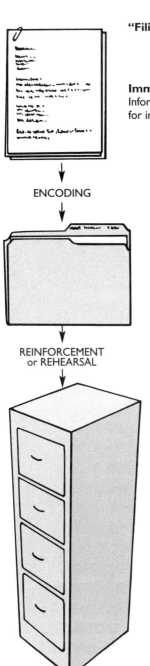

"Filing" a memory

Immediate or working memory
Information is received and noted, available
for immediate recall only

ENCODING

Short-term memory
The information is stored and available
for recall over minutes or hours

REINFORCEMENT
or REHEARSAL

Long-term memory
The information is stored as a fairly
permanent record

information. This is equivalent to the formation of a short-term memory; the pieces of information have been encoded into a finite package that is available for retrieval.

The secretary may then decide to take the labeled file (the short-term memory) and slot it into an appropriate place in a filing cabinet. This is equivalent to the formation of a long-term memory.

Sometime later, when the information is needed, a search is initiated. The file cabinet is opened, the drawer pulled out and the labels of various files (or memories) are scanned until the correct one is found. The file is then lifted out as a unit, brought to the desk and opened, and the information is examined and used. This is the equivalent of a memory being recalled.

People with Alzheimer's disease have difficulty with all phases of this process, but especially with the creation of new memories (learning). To pursue the office analogy, they have difficulty making up new files and encoding them properly. The examination of existing files, once retrieved and spread out on the desk, is often well preserved.

Of course, our memory function is a lot more complex than any filing cabinet. We can adjust or reorganize many files rapidly (picking out things that happened in the summer of 1954, or animals beginning with the letter *B*). Computers are very good at sorting information into different categories like this (a phenomenon known as *cross-referencing*) and assembling information from different memory banks into one new unit. People with Alzheimer's disease lose this ability to manipulate or reclassify memories. They are better at examining a single reinforced unit of memory stored in the long-term system.

The Neurology of Memory

No one knows exactly how memories are constructed, at a

microscopic level, within the brain, but it is thought that we form a memory by establishing a connection between neurons, creating a track, or flow of information, between brain cells. Imagine one neuron connecting with another, then another and another, like a string of Christmas lights. When all the cells connect, the memory has been constructed. The information has been encoded, or formed into a unit. It's as if the string of Christmas lights is now plugged in and has "lit up."

In immediate, or working, memory most tracks or connections between neurons are not permanent, and the information held in them quickly fades. We can repeat a list of unrelated numbers just after it's presented to us, but we will have forgotten it in two or three hours unless we process the numbers to a different stage of memory. If the information is trivial, we allow the mind to clear the track—we actually choose to forget the numbers. However, we recognize other information as being important to us, and so we preserve it by reinforcing the tracks—the connections—between the cells in the brain. We do this by incorporating the tracks into short-term (and eventually long-term) memory. At a microscopic level, these tracks or connections between cells do not easily fade.

A memory track that is frequently recalled or reinforced is much more firmly established in the brain than one that is not. The use of the information again and again in daily life bolsters the pattern in the brain. It's as if the pattern of connections between neurons becomes stronger with repetitive use—the track becomes "etched" more deeply in the brain each time. We know that the connections between neurons are mediated through chemical transmitters—neurotransmitters—and that the more frequently the neurons connect chemically, the more prepared they are to connect again. This phenomenon is called "facilitation." We "learned" lists of information at school this way, repeating the components again and again until the information was well established within the brain and could be recalled at will. Information that has been in the brain for a long time and has been recalled often is more easily brought back to use.

Short-Term Memory Lost Early

Unfortunately, one of the first areas of the brain damaged by Alzheimer's disease is the one that controls short-term memory. This area is in the temporal lobe of the cortex, in what is called the *hippocampus*. (*Hippocampus* is Latin for "sea horse"; to early anatomists the shape of the area suggested this tiny sea creature.) No one knows why the hippocampus is so severely damaged early in the disease, when much of the rest of the brain seems unaffected. However, changes in this area of the brain can be seen on CT scans as the first objective physical sign of the disease process.

Because the ability to form short-term memories is an essential link in learning information, and because the hippocampus is severely damaged early in Alzheimer's disease, people with Alzheimer's have great difficulty in learning new information—that is, in transferring it from immediate memory into long-term. They are able to repeat a list of words to you, using their intact immediate-memory skills, just as accurately as a healthy person would. They are also able to call up long-term memories—well-established memories held in a relatively intact area in the brain—without difficulty. However, the critical middle step of forming a short-term memory—the step that occurs in the damaged hippocampus—is significantly impaired, and they will remember few of the words in the list if you ask them to repeat it several minutes or hours later.

Physical Memory

So far we have been speaking of intellectual memory—the ability to recall learned information. But there is another kind of memory, a deeper and different kind, called "physical memory." We are able to learn complex physical tasks through repetition and study. We can teach our bodies to move in a particular way for a desired purpose, such as dancing, playing the piano or riding a bicycle. In each of these examples of learned physical behavior, we have integrated complicated bodily actions into a fluid sequence, with one action following another. Repetition of the sequence establishes the physical activity as a memory to be recalled at will. At a microscopic level, a track has been formed between neurons in the brain, and initiation of the memory causes the track to "light up" like the string of Christmas lights.

The training of athletes is based in large part on this learning of physical behavior, but it applies to the rest of us as well. Typing, knitting, driving an automobile, even shuffling playing-cards or tying our shoes are all examples of physical memories. Like intellectual memories, they are reinforced by repetition, so that the actions may reach the point of being done "automatically." You don't actively consider how your hands should move when you tie your shoes—you just do it. In doing so you are calling forth from your brain a packet of information about an orderly progression of physical activities—a physical memory. The centers that control physical movement are located in a different area of the brain from the centers that control thought, and this anatomical difference is once again important in Alzheimer's. Early in the disease the areas that control physical movement remain relatively undamaged, so that many physical memories are well preserved in people whose intellectual abilities are severely affected. Thus, someone may be able to play the piano well, long after forgetting the names of the pieces being played.

Retrieval of Memories

Once a packet of information enters the mind as a memory, it is available for retrieval or recall. Unimportant information stored in working memory will be forgotten very quickly unless it is processed into short-term memory. Information in short-term memory can be retrieved at will over a much longer period of time, often days or weeks, and information in long-term memory may be retrievable over a lifetime.

The retrieval of any memory is impaired by stress or anxiety. We all know this from experience: it's much more difficult to recall details—such as a person's name—when we are nervous or under pressure. In Alzheimer's disease, insecurity and stress often affect the retrieval of a particular memory. This is why people with Alzheimer's can sometimes remember something in a relaxed situation, but not when they are agitated or disturbed.

Forgetfulness Can Be Normal

Some loss of memory facility is an inevitable consequence of normal aging. We all eventually struggle to remember names, where we set down the keys, whether we locked the door when we left in the morning. This "benign forgetfulness" differs markedly from the memory loss of Alzheimer's, in many ways.

We know that to be formed into a memory, a piece of information must be seen as significant; it has to be identified as different from any similar information we have been presented with before, and once it has been encoded into a memory, it has to be reinforced frequently in order to be recalled at will. In normal aging the process of encoding is often the cause of minor memory problems: we simply don't register something as worthy of being remembered, so the encoding process is not completed correctly and the information is lost.

Imagine you are late one morning, and you've hurried through your shower and dressing. You have a fast cup of coffee in the kitchen and head for the door. As you open the door you remember that you have to take your briefcase to work, so you rush back inside and get it. Outside, you suddenly wonder if you turned off the burner underneath the coffeepot. You climb into the car uncertain of the answer, but eventually, not trusting your memory, you go back to make sure. The act of turning off the burner was simply not significant enough, in the hurry of the morning, to be encoded.

Our senses are constantly being bombarded with information and we can't possibly notice every single event or fact presented to us, so we choose the important ones. The first step in forming a memory is the active choice of deciding if something is worth remembering. "Where did I put my keys?" is a common question as we age because we failed to recognize that the place we set the keys down a few minutes earlier was worthy of note—that is, was worthy of forming a new memory track. This is not true memory loss but absentmindedness—failure to focus on the event. We have set down the keys thousands of times in our lives, and nothing was unique enough about the last time to make us notice it.

However, we have no trouble in recognizing significant events as being noteworthy. It is quite common and normal to forget where you parked your car at the mall—one comic referred to this as "Mallzheimer's disease." But we would be quite certain that we brought the car, that we stopped for gas, that we were hurrying to get to the store before closing time and so on. People with Alzheimer's disease might forget not only where the car was, but whether they'd brought it or why they'd gone to the store in the first place. Eighty percent of seniors complain of some decrease in memory, but the memory loss is qualitatively different from that seen in Alzheimer's disease; it doesn't apply to significant events, and it can usually be remedied by ensuring that the information is properly encoded—that is, by identifying what needs to be remembered, focusing on it as being important and then reinforcing it.

Seniors Need More Time

As a general rule, processing time is longer in older people than it is in younger people; the manipulation of information takes longer. It takes older people more time to memorize something (that is, to form a long-term memory) and more time to use information in reasoning or calculating. Encoding becomes poorer—less information can be registered at one time as we age—and we are also more easily distracted. Seniors need to focus more on the uniqueness of an event (especially an often-repeated one such as turning off the stove) to make it a memory. Memory processes also take more energy; seniors have to work harder at forming a memory, and at such things as comparison, deduction and interpretation. However, the conclusions they draw from this manipulation of information are just as accurate as those of the young. In addition, their wealth of experience allows them to see the problem from a different perspective; seniors may take longer to answer, but their answer is worth waiting for.

Though the amount of information we can hold in short-term memory decreases with age, the amount held in long-term memory increases dramatically—chiefly because seniors have so much experience. In many traditional societies this expanse of long-term memory is recognized as the "wisdom of the elders." Unfortunately, the retrieval of this information is not as rapid or dependable as it was in youth. This explains the

Memory changes with normal aging

Absentmindedness: As we age, we need to pay more attention to anything we wish to encode into short-term memory; we must concentrate on it. It takes more energy and more focus to encode information, and lack of this focus is the commonest cause of poor memory in the aged.

Decreased reserve: Short-term memory has a finite capacity, and as we age the capacity becomes smaller. Many young people can hold nine or ten unrelated digits in short-term memory. Most seniors can hold only five or six.

Increased processing time: As we age, we need longer to encode a memory, and more rehearsal or repetition. If the memory can be tied to previous experience, this processing time is significantly shorter.

Partial recall: Our ability to recall information is preserved well with age. However, the recall is often not total—we may have something "on the tip of the tongue," even though we can identify other important characteristics of the memory.

Memory changes in Alzheimer's disease

Immediate memory: There is little change early in the course of the disease.

Short-term memory: This is usually affected very early in the disease, and is often the first hint of any trouble in the brain.

Inability to learn: Learning depends on short-term memory, so early in the disease people are unable to incorporate new information.

Long-term memory: These stores are often well maintained, especially early in the disease. Eventually they fail as well.

frustratingly common phenomenon of having something "on the tip of your tongue." You are quite aware that you know the information requested, but your recall isn't able to bring it to your consciousness. Often, pursuing the information from a different direction is all that's needed. (If you can't remember what you planned for dinner, for example, try remembering what groceries you bought.) The stress and frustration of not being able to remember frequently make the process even less reliable. In another setting, at another time, the information may come to your mind without delay.

Benign forgetfulness versus the memory loss of Alzheimer's

Benign forgetfulness
- usually inconsequential details, such as the names of distant acquaintances
- not associated with other neurological problems, such as difficulties with reasoning, arithmetic, language
- often the information can be recalled later, usually in complete detail
- fully aware of not being able to recall, and often quite troubled by it
- spotty, inconsistent memory loss, usually worse with stress or pressure
- can remember anything if it is focused on and learned
- memory loss easily remedied by prompting (making lists, giving clues and so on)
- is often frustrating and irritating but never interferes significantly with social and professional activities
- what is the last thing you forgot? If you can recall full details of the event, you probably don't have Alzheimer's disease

Alzheimer's
- often significant details such as grandchildren's names
- always associated with decreased ability to reason and calculate
- often the information is simply gone, unable to be recalled, and prompting does not help
- often seemingly indifferent—"It's not important" or "I don't need to know that" are common reactions
- diffuse decrease in memory for all events, particularly recently learned information
- ability to learn new information—no matter how much it's focused upon—is markedly restricted. Immediate recall is normal, but recall hours to days later is not
- Alzheimer's sufferers not only lose the list, they forget they made one
- interferes significantly with social and professional activities
- even the act of forgetting is forgotten. The person is unaware (cannot remember) that there was a problem at all

Test yourself. If you can learn the names of ten objects and repeat them in ten minutes, your memory is probably normal.

Mild Cognitive Impairment

Alzheimer's disease is a slow, progressive disease that first appears as short-term memory loss. Later, other cognitive functions, personality and judgment are affected. It is very difficult to pinpoint when the disease first began—but it is clear now that the memory loss may have started many years before diagnosis was made. Usually, by the time the diagnosis is apparent and the memory loss is obvious, significant damage has already been done to the brain.

Ideally, we would like to identify people who have just developed Alzheimer's, to treat the disorder as early as possible. Research has now identified some characteristics of people whose memory loss is greater than that seen in normal older adults (more than benign forgetfulness) but not severe enough to qualify as Alzheimer's disease. These individuals have *mild cognitive impairment*. They are usually more forgetful than they were in the past, and more forgetful than expected for their age and education. In most cases this condition is likely a *prodromal*, or very early, state of Alzheimer's disease. These are the characteristics:

- memory complaint
- a family member or friend who confirms that there is progressive memory loss
- more memory loss than others of similar age and education
- thinking and reasoning normal apart from the memory loss
- normal functioning in activities of daily living
- no dementia

When people with these characteristics are followed up over time, about 6 to 12 percent develop Alzheimer's disease every year. Currently, there are many studies underway to try to target such people, and to examine a variety of strategies to prevent them from developing Alzheimer's disease.

While attempts are being made to identify people just before they develop Alzheimer's, and those who are in the very early stages, researchers are also working to develop treatments that will improve the symptoms of memory loss at these early stages. Drugs like tacrine, donepezil, rivastigmine and galan-tamine are being used in an attempt to improve the memory loss. Other components like antioxidants (vitamin E), anti-inflammatory agents, hormones (estrogen), secretase inhibitors and immunotherapy are being tested in the very early stages of the disease, to prevent further progression.

Memory Loss Interferes with Life

Sooner or later, the memory defects of Alzheimer's disease begin to interfere with the person's social and professional life. Obviously a small amount of memory difficulty would inter-fere with the work of an accountant or a pharmacist much earlier than with that of a laborer, but it's characteristic that in Alzheimer's disease the memory impairment is significant enough to interfere with daily activities. This is in marked con-trast to the memory loss that occurs with normal aging, which usually applies to only inconsequential details.

In addition, the memory loss in Alzheimer's disease never appears by itself; it's always part of a larger picture of cogni-tive decline, of loss of the other faculties of thinking, such as reasoning and calculating. Alzheimer's disease is diagnosed not by memory loss alone, but by significant memory loss asso-ciated with evidence of impairment of other brain functions. In other words, the memory loss in Alzheimer's is evidence of generalized brain failure.

Forgetting How to Learn

In early Alzheimer's disease, quite a common problem is that people lose the ability to learn. They are no longer able to incorporate new information into their behavior because their ability to form short-term memories—which is essential to learning—has been damaged. They may function well at home, within the confines of their own house, but if they find themselves in a strange place—perhaps in a hotel or unfamiliar house—they become agitated and confused, even unable to function. They have been using long-term memory to navigate at home, but now they need short-term memory to learn the new layout. They simply don't have the ability to learn this new information.

Language Changes in Alzheimer's Disease

For years, preaching in the isolated communities of the British Columbia coast, the Reverend Mr. O'Malley had been known for the passion of his sermons. He was a large and powerful man with a superb speaking style, and few of his parishioners left his services without being moved by the conviction and eloquence of this energetic Irishman. He was still active in the church in his late seventies, when his wife noticed that his sermons were slowly changing. Though the reverend could still quote extended passages from the Scriptures with the same accuracy and zeal as in his youth, she noted that he sometimes lost the thread of the sermon, the flow and purpose of it. Sometimes he stopped in midsentence, apparently unable to complete his thought. He would look confused, as if trying to recall where he was. But he was still able to finish the service with the familiar phrasing and ritual of the church, and he warmly greeted his parishioners at the door as usual.

The reverend found it necessary to retire at last when he was 78, and he was diagnosed with Alzheimer's disease soon afterward. Curiously, it was his most precious ability, his power to move people with his speech, that was most affected by the disease. Exchanging pleasantries, he was perfectly normal and completely at ease, but if he was pressed for details in a conversation he easily became upset, and often he would hesitate, as if unable to recall the proper words.

In the office he greeted the doctor warmly and shook his hand with a reassuring strength. The conversation, though, was quite abnormal:

Doctor: So, Reverend, how are you doing today?

Reverend: I am well, Doctor, and how is the world treating you?

Doctor: I'm well as well. Tell me, how does it feel to be retired?

Reverend: Well, ah … retired … I'm not really the same … you know … as before … not with churchgoers or ah … mainly at home … with my Mary … not the usual …

Doctor: You've had a long career of preaching on the coast. Tell me about it.

Reverend: Well, it was wonderful in the service of God over the years … many years in the church … with sermons and visiting … but now …

Though the power was still in his words, his meaning was not always obvious, and the Reverend Mr. O'Malley would turn to his wife for help in completing the phrases.

Over the next year and a half the reverend worsened at home, became combative with his wife and, on several occasions, became quite agitated when he mistakenly thought his wife was an intruder. Eventually, after weeks of his nightly episodes of wandering, she found it necessary to admit him to a nursing home. He was still able to recall phrases from the Bible, and delighted the nursing staff with extended quotations from the Scriptures, correctly reciting the particulars of both chapter and verse. However, his other language skills worsened markedly. When the doctor visited, he was greeted warmly by the priest in the usual enthusiastic manner, but the conversation quickly deteriorated:

Reverend: Well, Doctor, how are you doing this fine morning?

Doctor: Just fine, Reverend—and you?

Reverend: With the Lord's grace, enjoying this fine morning.

Doctor: How are things at the nursing home here?

Reverend: Well, things … are … where?

Doctor: Here at the nursing home.

Reverend: Well, I think things are … fulfilling … this fine morning.

Doctor: Fulfilling? What do you mean?

Reverend: Well, I think that's what may be … sometimes.

Doctor: Are you happy here?

Reverend: Happy here … well, for many times … things are …fulfilling.

As time passed, the priest's speech slowly worsened to the point where he was unable to construct a complete sentence and often repeated a phrase or two from the question put to him. Sometimes he just didn't seem to understand the purpose of the words, though they were repeated for him and he was able to say them back mechanically. Nurses would ask if he wanted to have his bath now, and he would repeat the phrase "bath now" to them as if he understood. However, when they poured water into the bathtub and began to undress him he became quite agitated, as if surprised by the whole event.

Many times he repeated the phrase "yes, amen" as part of his conversation, but even this became less frequent as he worsened. Yet he was still able to greet the doctor, and indeed many of his fellow patients, with warmth and affection, just as he had done for years in the church.

Eventually, after three years in the nursing home, he lost the ability to participate in any conversation in a meaningful way. His ability to communicate was limited to very simple words such as "no," and he did not speak spontaneously at all, except on rare occasions when he would cry out a simple phrase such as "oh, God" for no apparent reason. For the last six months of his life in the nursing home, the Reverend Mr. O'Malley was unable to speak at all; one of his most precious abilities was entirely denied him.

Language: A Precious Gift

Communicating thoughts and feelings by means of vocal sounds is one of the most prized and individual of human abilities. As a species, we developed this special skill because we are social creatures, interdependent and thus necessarily cooperative. Language allows us to live with others. It gives us the ability to share our needs, our desires, our aspirations. It enables us to be intimate. We can, of course, communicate in other ways, but without language our human existence is much poorer—we become isolated and detached, deprived of one of the joys of life. Unfortunately, deterioration in language is always part of Alzheimer's disease.

The Neurology of Language

The phenomenon of language is complex and involves many different areas of the brain in association or communication. When we are asked a simple question such as "How are you today?" we hear the words in our ears, but the impulses created by vibration of the eardrum travel into the area of the brain that specializes in the reception of sounds, located in the temporal lobe. Here the impulses are translated into recognizable words, which are then reassembled into a meaningful pattern. This transformation, usually done on the left side of the brain, gives us a reasonable understanding of the question. The next step occurs in another area of our brain, the frontal lobe, where we begin to analyze the question and choose a response. Once this is done, the frontal lobe sends impulses to yet another area in the brain, the motor cortex, to initiate impulses from this area to begin to form a reply. From the motor cortex the impulses travel to the muscles of articulation in the mouth and throat, and a specific reply—"I'm fine, thank you. How are you?"—is expressed. The processing of the original question and the formation of a response involve several areas of the brain communicating with one another. We take these communications for granted, and of course the whole process requires only a fraction of a second, but these association areas—the pathways between specific sites in the brain—are severely affected by Alzheimer's disease.

How Language Changes First Appear

The changes may be subtle to begin with. One of the first is an inability to find exactly the right word—a medical condition called *anomia* (from the Latin meaning "without a name")—and it is thought to be a phenomenon of memory. Instead of saying "coffee cup," the person may say "the thing to hold coffee." "Key" becomes "door opener" and "toothbrush" becomes "tooth cleaner." Often, in the early stages, people are still able to explain what they mean—to communicate an understanding without actually using the specific word, a technique called *circumlocution* (literally, "talking around it"). It's the same trick we often use when we're learning a second language—we may not know the precise word for something in the foreign language, but we can describe it well enough that our meaning becomes apparent. The first Alzheimer's patient, Auguste D., was unable to remember the word "cup" but referred to the item as a "milk jug." Anomia seems to occur at first only with objects the person doesn't often see or use, but later occurs with common objects.

Simple errors are common, especially in words that sound alike—"cup of tea" may become "cup of tie." The grouping of words by category becomes impaired, because this function demands "refiling" of groups of objects within the mind and thus requires a degree of reasoning that is often lost early in Alzheimer's disease. For example, listing animals that begin with the letter *A*, or pieces of furniture made with wood, is likely to be difficult or impossible for someone with Alzheimer's.

Lost Meanings

Comprehension of language also becomes impaired as the disease progresses, and so people become more insecure during conversations and reluctant to engage in any but the most superficial discourse. The output of both written and spoken language decreases, and reading becomes less frequent and enjoyable. People are often well aware they can't find the right words, and deliberately avoid situations where their language will be put to the test. Friends and relatives may notice an inability to find the appropriate word, and grammatical errors and other difficulties may result in half-finished sentences or ideas being filled in by the listener. Others often don't appreciate how little the person understands what has been said. The pathways that give meaning to the collections of words we know as language have been damaged to the point where the person can no longer fully grasp the sense of the phrases and sentences. This is why many people with Alzheimer's are unable to participate in conversation, or obey simple commands. They have heard the words (that part of their brain is working well), but the interconnected pathways that should allow processing of the information into a conscious response have been damaged. They listen to the conversation and try to participate, but they are unable to do so completely. Though they can hear, they cannot correctly understand what is being said, nor can they form a plan of action to respond to the information.

Thus hampered, but wanting to continue attempts at communication, they may use repetitive, superficial, meaningless phrases such as "Well, this is it" or "Right on." These phrases are usually ones they have employed for years, and they are employed now just to keep the conversation going. Questions are often repeated as the person struggles to understand what is being asked. The problem is reinforced when short-term-memory damage prevents the person from remembering the last time the question was asked.

Surprisingly, superficial conversation is often remarkably well preserved. The simple pleasantries of daily life—greetings and farewells, inconsequential discussions of nonspecifics—are often quite normal until Alzheimer's disease is well advanced. This results in fairly normal superficial contact with people whose language abilities are significantly damaged. A casual meeting with such a person may reveal no evidence of language disorder—in fact, the communication may be perfectly normal. Only with a more complex exchange do the defects become obvious. This is because such perfunctory encounters have been repeated many times throughout the person's life and have thus been well learned; they are long-term memories and do not call for any reasoning or cognitive power. They are often accompanied by the familiar physical signs of communication—shaking hands or reaching out for a touch—and the appropriate facial expressions. Those who have enjoyed contact with others throughout their lives frequently have their social language skills well preserved long into the disease.

Communication in Late Alzheimer's Disease

As the disease progresses, language deteriorates further. Incomplete sentences and rambling patterns of words replace coherent speech, though articulation, the actual ability to form the sounds and words, remains intact. Comprehension of others'

Conversation and speech changes in Alzheimer's disease

Initial stage

- anomia—difficulty in finding the correct word
- circumlocution—talking around the word that can't be recalled
- withdrawing from complicated or intellectual conversations
- substituting similar words for the right one, or words that sound almost the same

Middle stage

- using more empty phrases and words—"That's right," "Right on"
- avoiding conversation, decreased initiative in speech
- forgetting grammar and sentence construction
- losing train of thought during conversation
- losing pleasure in reading and writing
- repeating phrases within sentences
- leaving sentences unfinished
- sometimes not seeming to understand meaning

Late stage

- rarely initiating conversation
- not following simple commands—not understanding
- being unable to read
- being unable to write
- repeating single words or short meaningless phrases such as "Okay" or "No, no, no"
- rambling when speaking, being unable to follow a train of thought
- echolalia or paralalia (repeating part or all of the question asked, as an answer)
- eventually, speaking unintelligibly (grunting)
- in terminal phase, becoming mute

speech becomes even more abnormal—people simply *cannot* understand or act on the information being presented to them, even though they hear it. Though they can make some attempt at reply, the purpose of language (to transfer an idea from one person to another) is completely lost to them. This is why, later in the disease, people often seem to be ignoring their caregivers, or acting in a particular way just to spite them.

Sometimes words are repeated endlessly, or a word or phrase in the question is echoed to the questioner again and again, a phenomenon called *echolalia*. Occasionally an offensive word or phrase is repeated in this manner, causing great disturbance to those within earshot. It is important to understand that the meaning of such words or phrases is lost to the person—the formation of the sounds is caused by the disease process producing a "short circuit" in the language area. The language itself has no message or implication. It's also important to accept the fact that these are not voluntary phenomena. They are completely out of the person's control, and reflect the lack of connection between various areas of the brain.

Finally all significant verbal communication ceases, and people become mute, totally isolated and turned in on themselves, unable to convey any feeling or thought process by language. Like Auguste D., they die without a word.

Loss of Judgment and Reasoning Ability

The Stranger Within

For years, Roy had enjoyed the respect of the community where he lived. He worked as the only pharmacist in a small-town drugstore that his father had built, and had the privilege of being able to help many, many people through his profession. He greeted each and every one of his friends and customers by name in a confident and avuncular manner from behind the counter.

He was devastated when, after a series of glaring errors in prescriptions, his family doctor, an old friend, told Roy he had Alzheimer's disease. Roy had noticed that he just couldn't seem to keep up with all the new drugs coming onto the market; he found it very difficult to keep them straight in his mind. He had to make extensive notes whenever one of the drug reps visited the pharmacy with a new product. For a year or two he'd been having the drug dosages checked by his assistant "just to be sure"—and it was becoming more and more common for the assistant, a young woman with no formal pharmacology training, to change the dosage because of an error. Soon the errors became so frequent that Roy was simply overwhelmed—confused and unable to cope with the complexity of the job he had loved for so long.

All this was very disturbing to Roy, but in addition he had noticed that he was losing one of his most prized abilities: he could no longer recognize his faithful customers, no longer greet them by their first names in the manner that had given him so much pleasure all his life. Many of the newer customers—those who had only recently begun frequenting his drugstore—he claimed he'd never seen before in his life. Tragically, he didn't seem able to recognize even some of his most trusted friends and long-term associates. He forgot their names, or appeared indifferent when they greeted him in the store.

Roy retired, professing that he was just "too old," but he was ashamed of his losses, and though he still owned the drugstore, he found it too disturbing to visit there—he couldn't even remember the names of his employees. Once, an embarrassing altercation took place when he confronted the young delivery boy, insisting that the boy was an impostor and demanding that the police be called in.

But the worst episode of confusion occurred at home.

One day after a shower, Roy rushed downstairs, still dripping wet and dressed only in a bath towel. He was very agitated and screamed at his poor wife, "Come quickly, Dee. There's a burglar upstairs!"

She wanted to call the police, but he insisted on taking her by the hand and together, even though she knew it was dangerous, they snuck up the stairs to the bathroom. Roy motioned to her that the burglar was inside. He opened the bathroom door carefully, but his terrified wife couldn't see anyone in the small room.

"There's no one here, Roy," she said with relief.

"Look!" said Roy, shaking with fear as he pointed toward the large mirror over the sink in front of them. "There he is! He's right beside you!"

Roy's startled wife looked where he was pointing, but all she could see was her own reflection in the mirror, next to her wide-eyed husband's.

Then, in a sickening moment, she understood. Roy didn't recognize himself. He thought the image staring back at him was that of an intruder, someone he had never seen before, a burglar in the sanctity of their home.

She slowly led Roy out of the bathroom and tried to calm him. He couldn't understand why she was crying but wouldn't let him go back into the bathroom to confront the stranger in their home.

Stranger in a Strange World

One of the most disabling signs of Alzheimer's disease is loss of the ability to identify everyday objects and their uses. This medical phenomenon is called *agnosia* (the word is derived from the Greek and means "without knowledge") and it is behind many of the bewildering behaviors seen in the disease. For example, a woman is shown a hairbrush after a bath and can neither recognize it as something she has seen before nor use it appropriately. The look and feel of the hairbrush do not trigger an understanding of what the object is or what it's used for. Vision and touch remain intact within the brain; what has been damaged is the ability to put these sensory inputs together into a concept of an object recognized as a hairbrush. She simply can't do it, because the areas in the brain connecting those sensory inputs have been damaged. Sitting beside the bath with the unrecognizable object in her hand, the woman is bewildered and confused.

Sometimes agnosia results in someone "recognizing" an object incorrectly—often confusing it with something similar in use and function. The hairbrush is incorrectly thought to be a toothbrush—with devastating results when toothpaste is spread over it!

Agnosia applies to people as well as objects, and causes much of the heartache of the disease. Just as those with Alzheimer's sometimes can't identify such common objects as hairbrushes, they may also become unable to recognize family and friends because of a combination of memory loss and damage to the connecting pathways within the brain. At first they can't identify people they haven't seen for a long time, but as the disease progresses, further damage within the brain results in their being unable to identify even those who have been close to them throughout their lives. Faces of siblings, business partners and close friends no longer evoke a smile of recognition, a lifting up of the face in greeting. Instead they seem barely to recognize that their old friends are in the room, and the friends are deeply pained by this. Sometimes there is a hint of acknowledgment—the friend is recognized at one level, but the person with Alzheimer's is unable to complete the association by recalling the name or particulars. Eventually, no matter how much contact has gone before, how much love has flowed between them, the person with Alzheimer's doesn't recognize even children or spouse. The most important people in the victim's life are greeted with indifference, with a vacancy that is heart-rending in its sadness.

This agnosia regarding other people also applies to the individuals themselves. They stop being able to identify themselves. Roy's misinterpretation of his image in the mirror is a good example; within his brain he was unable to construct a correct image of himself and then recognize it in the mirror.

Understanding Agnosia

We know that certain areas of the brain are severely affected early in Alzheimer's disease, while others are relatively spared. Unfortunately, the pathways that link various centers within the brain are often damaged quickly, so that specific parts of the brain can no longer communicate with other parts, even though they themselves may function relatively normally. Much as our cities are interconnected by highways, telephones and satellite hook-ups, so the various centers in the brain are interconnected through neural pathways that transmit information instantaneously. Thus, the speech center in the left temporal lobe knows what the visual center in the occipital lobe is "seeing" and what the emotional center in the limbic system is "feeling." Damage to these interconnecting pathways isolates these centers so that they cannot receive input from other centers, or influence one another. They have stopped "talking." A man with Alzheimer's disease is given a fork, and his sensory center recognizes it as something he has seen before, but with the pathways damaged he cannot tell you the name of the object he is holding, and he has absolutely no idea what it's used for or how he should hold it. He can no longer use his brain as a whole to manipulate or correlate information and feelings. Simple arithmetic such as that used in checking a bank balance becomes impossible. Playing cards is no longer pleasant. Keeping score in golf or bridge, organizing the day's medicines, counting change at the grocery store—all these tasks become much more difficult, and eventually impossible. Sequential tasks such as setting the table or cooking from a recipe are also too much. Even the relatively simple consecutive actions needed to take a bath (run the water, adjust the temperature, remove clothes one at a time, wash, dry and so on) are too complicated when areas in the brain are separated from one another.

Damage to these same pathways prevents people with early Alzheimer's disease from properly integrating new information within the brain. Though the listening center may hear a question, there is no connection to the area of insight that could formulate a reasonable response based on experience. The visual center may "see" a person moving in the bedroom mirror, but the judgment center is not consulted to see if the image is recognizable. A wife visits at the nursing home and a genuine warmth is felt from her presence, yet the husband doesn't really understand who it is sitting beside him, holding his hand with such gentleness and compassion.

Forgetting How

Apraxia (from the Greek for "not acting") is another commonly seen sign of Alzheimer's disease. It's the inability to carry out purposeful movements and actions despite intact motor and sensory systems. It is often present quite early in Alzheimer's disease but may not be recognized. It can be the cause of much frustration for caregivers who fail to understand that those they are caring for have lost the mental ability to complete everyday activities. Such basic physical acts as eating, walking and even dressing—the more automatic tasks of life— are usually not a problem at first, but the more technical tasks are. The person may no longer be able to operate a remote control for the television, or set the temperature of the oven for baking. An organizational task such as creating a grocery list may be impossible. Ominously, the reasoning that is so important in financial matters begins to fail, and errors inevitably appear. Minor chores that were easily accomplished before become extremely difficult. As time goes by, even simpler activities become affected, and the person has difficulty dressing and eating. He or she is physically able to put on socks and shoes or lift a fork to the mouth, but mentally these purposeful movements can no longer be carried out sequentially. Bowel and bladder needs cannot be handled, and accidents result. The person has no voluntary control over this inability, and is *not* doing it on purpose to create problems or get attention. He or she has simply lost the reasoning power to be able to see the task through to completion.

Self-Neglect

An inability to reason, to draw conclusions from observations and use correct judgment, is always present in Alzheimer's disease. This, combined with memory changes and apraxia, is manifested in serious cognitive errors—such as paying the same bill four times or leaving the house for a walk in midwinter with only light clothing on. It is the reasoning ability, the facility to evaluate information and make a correct decision, that is the problem. Self-neglect often follows; people no longer take pride in their appearance or clothing and become slovenly. They also become careless, and this carelessness often threatens their safety. It is common to find irons still on, kettles boiled dry, cigarettes left burning, dishwashers improperly loaded and so on. These errors result from a combination of deficits: loss of memory, apraxia, agnosia and loss of basic reasoning power.

Moreover, since these people are also unable to process new information, to form new memories, they no longer profit from their errors; they do not seem to learn from their mistakes. The compounding of all these deficits in brain function causes a repetition of the problems, day after day, week after week, as they suffer a slow but relentless decline in their ability to comprehend the world around them.

Spatial Disorientation

Another sign of early Alzheimer's disease is confusion or disorientation in fairly familiar surroundings. Typically, a person leaves home for an everyday task such as shopping or visiting a friend and becomes lost, despite having known the route well for years. Orientation in space demands a constant assimilation of data and a rapid processing of this information. We take it for granted. On the way to go shopping, for instance, we constantly check our environment to be sure we're on the right path, keeping our destination and purpose in mind, and making adaptations and adjustments as we progress. Once again, this requires the association of various areas of the brain; disparate centers must communicate with one another. This ability becomes disturbed early in the course of Alzheimer's. People get lost on familiar trips. At first disorientation occurs outside the home, but in time it occurs within the home itself.

Any change of environment is a significant challenge to most people with Alzheimer's. They simply cannot form a new visual map in their minds. This leads to extreme anxiety, and because of this, many people with Alzheimer's disease become less venturesome, less enthusiastic about traveling (especially by themselves), and instead prefer to spend their time in and around their homes. They become recluses, and this, in combination with their language and communication difficulties, reinforces their isolation.

Some idea of the magnitude of this spatial disorientation can be seen by studying drawings that people with Alzheimer's have made of clocks. Though the general idea of a clock is there, the particulars are usually wrong. The numbers are jumbled off to one side, or are only partly present, or have grossly obvious defects. People with Alzheimer's simply "see" the world differently than we do.

Behavioral and Personality Changes
In addition to the changes in memory and reasoning power

that are an integral part of the disease, people with Alzheimer's also develop changes in their behavior and personality. These changes are usually very upsetting to the family, because the person appears to be someone altogether different. People become unpredictable, childlike, sometimes even frightening, as they deteriorate. Their personalities, the way they respond in particular situations and to particular people, may change dramatically.

As with deterioration of memory and cognition, these changes occur because of specific damage to areas within the brain. Behavioral changes commonly seen include sleep disorders, hallucinations and delusions, disturbances in activity levels, aggression and mood disturbances.

**Examples of
clock drawings**

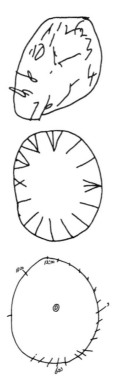

Sleep Disorders

Sleep is a wonderful but complicated process of daily rejuvenation. Good-quality sleep is necessary for our energy and mental well-being. Unfortunately, sleep quality deteriorates very early in the course of Alzheimer's disease, robbing people of its healing and comfort.

Sleep occurs in distinct stages. One of these stages, called "deep sleep," is the most refreshing, the one that produces the feeling of being well rested. People with Alzheimer's disease have markedly decreased amounts of deep sleep and thus are often quite tired; they feel that their sleep was not refreshing and that their minds are not clear. They also have multiple awakenings throughout the night and difficulty getting back to sleep. These changes are thought to be due to neuron damage and the loss of the connecting pathways in the brain that initiate sleep and maintain it throughout the night.

Sleep disturbances progress throughout the years of the disease, and are the most common reason families give for the decision to institutionalize their loved one. As the disease advances, people often have reversal of the normal sleep-wake cycle—they sleep off and on during the day and are awake at night. At home this may mean that the person naps most of the day but is up and about the house at night, turning lights on, perhaps beginning to cook breakfast, even trying to get out for a walk, and quite resistant to the idea of returning to bed. In the hospital it often means patients try to crawl out of bed over the side rails, try to get dressed, and disturb others.

Some researchers feel that decreased levels of melatonin are responsible for this pattern. Melatonin is a hormone produced in the pineal gland of the brain and it is secreted in the darkness of night. It prepares the cells of the brain and the rest of the body for sleep. In Alzheimer's disease this hormone secre-

Common sleep changes

- *Lack of deep sleep.* Sleep is much less refreshing and restorative; this is seen early in the disease.
- *Multiple awakenings with difficulty returning to sleep.* Normal adults awaken four or five times a night, but with Alzheimer's disease awakenings may total 15 or 20 a night.
- *Sleep not tied to darkness.* This often causes daytime napping and midnight rambling, or even complete reversal of the normal day-night cycle of sleep. In one study some Alzheimer's sufferers spent nearly 40 percent of their bedtime hours awake and 20 percent of their daytime hours asleep.
- *Sundowning.* This increasing confusion and agitation that comes with evening is seen in the middle stages of Alzheimer's disease and is often the reason people are institutionalized. As the disease progresses and sleep becomes even poorer, many people spend much of their time in a *semipermanent drowsy state*, drifting off to sleep if not stimulated. However, this sleep is not refreshing and they never feel well rested.

tion is markedly decreased, with the result that sleep is no longer tied to nighttime.

As the disease progresses, many people sleep most of the time, day and night, and often have to be awakened for meals. Their sleep, however, is only a light comalike state caused by the progressive cell damage within their brains.

Sundowning

A particularly severe form of behavioral disorder seen commonly in Alzheimer's disease, "sundowning" manifests itself in recurring bouts of confusion and agitation associated with the darkness of evening and night. The person may be quite docile during the daytime, easily directed and passive, but as nighttime approaches this behavior changes. He or she often becomes agitated and restless, perhaps calling out and wandering, and commonly has some sort of emotional disturbance such as fear, or perhaps perceptual problems such as hallucinations. Sundowners don't seem to be as aware of their environment as they were during the day, and their speech and reasoning are markedly worse. They may seem quite upset or nervous, or be very angry and resist any attempts to direct them or return them to bed. They may be very loud, screaming or cursing, and often have markedly increased activity, such as pacing or repetitive motions of picking at objects. They may attempt to leave home. In their confusion they may even strike out at caregivers and loved ones, or may accuse them of stealing things, or of keeping them inside against their will. The whole process is frightening to caregivers, as the sufferer cannot be reasoned with. Sundowning is thought to occur because of the poor sleep quality in Alzheimer's disease, combined with the neuron loss.

Hallucinations and Delusions

Hallucinations are apparent perceptions of sights, sounds and so on that are not really there, and they occur in at least 25 percent of people with Alzheimer's disease. The word "hallucination" comes from the Latin meaning "to wander in the mind," and though hallucinations may involve any of the five senses, in Alzheimer's they are usually visual—people "see things" that aren't there. These hallucinations occur because of neuron damage in the brain, and they are quite real to the person, who often cannot believe that you can't see them too. Normally we see because we receive signals of external objects through our eyes and this information from our retinas is transferred to the back of the brain, where a corresponding image is constructed. In Alzheimer's disease the image is produced within the brain itself, without any external source, and it is incorporated in what the eye is seeing at the time. Sometimes the hallucination is a misrepresentation of what is actually there—for example, a movement of the window curtain in a darkened bedroom is "seen" as an intruder. Naturally, the phenomenon is very disturbing to both the person involved and the caregiver. Alzheimer's hallucinations often include people, such as dead relatives coming to visit. Like dreams, the hallucinations almost always carry a significant emotional component. People are usually quite upset by the sight, as it triggers a response of fear, sadness, anger or whatever. They are also very upset when it becomes apparent that no one else can see what they are seeing. This often feeds their feeling of distrust or paranoia.

Delusions are another common problem in Alzheimer's, and occur in up to 75 percent of sufferers. They are simply mistaken beliefs, or judgments that are not reasonable. The word comes from the Latin meaning "to play false or deceive." Someone with a delusion vigorously holds on to a belief without reasonable evidence for the belief, and in spite of reasonable evidence to the contrary. Everyone else can see how inappropriate the belief is, but the person remains firmly convinced. In spite of profound memory loss, delusions are often held over long periods of time.

The delusions of people with Alzheimer's disease are remarkably similar, and are often paranoid in nature. For example, 40 percent have the suspicion that their spouses or caregivers are purposefully hiding or stealing objects, and 25 percent believe that they're being imprisoned in living quarters that are not their own. "Take me home," they command frequently, in spite of obvious evidence that they are already at home. Auguste D., Dr. Alzheimer's patient, had an inappropriate jealousy about her husband's supposed infidelity. Many sufferers believe that they are still working, or that dead relatives (especially parents) are alive. Some insist that their caregivers are in fact their mother or father. This may be because the caregiver has taken over many of the parental roles (such as feeding and dressing) that they remember from childhood. Often people believe that the characters on the television screen are real and that they are able to converse with them, or, like Roy, that the image in the mirror is not them but an intruder or impostor. In one specific delusion called "Capgras syndrome," a person believes that his or her spouse has been replaced by an identical impostor.

Obviously many of these delusions are painful for loved ones and family, as they question the unselfish love and trust that are the basis of their relationship.

Disturbances in Activity Levels

As the disease progresses, many people with Alzheimer's disease are unable to channel their energy in socially productive ways (such as going to work or cleaning the house) and are not able to organize the complex sequence of physical events required in many recreational activities, such as bicycling, lawn bowling, physical education classes and so on. It's not that the neurons *controlling* motor movements are damaged early in the disease—in fact, they are preserved until very late—but rather that the neurons *organizing* the sequencing of complicated motor events are affected. Thus, people with the disease have no appropriate outlet for their physical energy, and disturbances in activity are common. These people have all the frustration and anxiety of their condition with essentially normal motor power, but without the organization and direction of the higher centers in the brain. There are three common variants of altered physical-activity patterns.

Pacing. This is a driven type of walking. People seem to be in a hurry, as if they're going somewhere with determination. Often they have an understanding of purpose—"I'm going home"—and frequently an intensity of emotion accompanies it—"I've got to go *now*." They cannot easily be prevented from walking, or distracted once they begin, though the pattern is usually circular and the destination is never reached.

Wandering. This is a more purposeless, relaxed kind of walking. People ramble from room to room. Sometimes they appear to be looking for something, though they are not always aware of what the "lost object" is. This pattern of activity may be associated with delusions such as searching for something lost or for a family member, and when it is, it may be accompanied by considerable anxiety.

Repetitive purposeful movements. People frequently repeat simple activities again and again—such as straightening out the contents of a drawer, smoothing flat and patting down the edge of a tablecloth or bed, folding and unfolding a handkerchief or writing incomprehensible letters in a notebook. There is a certain superficial purpose or driving force behind these activities (the person just *has* to do it), but the thought often cannot be fulfilled. The combination of memory loss and delusion contributes to this behavior, and the incessant repetition of questions or statements is annoying and frustrating to the caregiver. Sometimes this type of behavior (such as continual rubbing or washing of hands) is even damaging, and it can be very difficult to contain. Again the person is not easily distracted from the repetitive movements; it's as if the command to perform these activities is very strong and must be obeyed.

Aggression

Unfortunately, many people with Alzheimer's become aggressive during the course of their disease. They may have had a tendency to this trait before they became ill, but often it is a totally inappropriate quality that greatly disturbs their caregivers. The aggression reflects the diffuse neuron loss causing changes in the person's personality and emotional-control mechanisms. The aggressiveness is not willful or even within

You're not alone

In many communities, help is available from "friendly visitors"—people who come to your home, as volunteers or employees of an Alzheimer's association, just to sit and talk, or perhaps take the person with Alzheimer's for a walk. Their sympathetic presence is a welcome break for caregivers, and a pleasant distraction for the person with the disease. Many of these visitors are also very knowledgeable and experienced with regard to Alzheimer's.

Ask your local association about this program, and also about the Wandering Person Registry—a system of photo identification carried by the person with Alzheimer's and kept on file by the police, so that someone who wanders away can quickly be found and brought home.

the person's control; it simply reflects illness in the area of the brain that normally keeps anger and rage within limits.

Verbal abuse is common, and these outbursts often come as a result of the frustration of being unable to communicate in a particular situation. Cursing or the use of foul language is frequent and may be unceasing. Sometimes nonsensical words or syllables are shouted angrily over and over, reflecting damage to the language centers.

Physical aggression occurs in 25 percent of cases, and may consist of striking the caregiver, biting, scratching, slapping, pinching or grabbing. When caregivers suffer physical aggression it is always psychologically wounding to them.

A different kind of aggression, that of negativity, is seen in some people, who actively resist being bathed, being dressed, being toileted and so on.

Catastrophic Reaction

A particularly difficult form of aggression is the "catastrophic reaction." This is a severe outburst of anger and aggression resulting from a seemingly trivial request or situation. The response is inappropriately emotional, and consists of shouting, physical aggression and rage, often as a result of the person's inability to cope with his or her emotional reaction to the situation. Uncontrollable crying, extreme agitation, combativeness or temper tantrums may be seen as a response to such unmanageable circumstances.

Catastrophic reactions may take place in the context of a regular activity, such as bathing, but are more frequent when the person's mood has already been made more unstable by sudden changes in the environment, such as admission to the hospital, or other stress factors. Anger or frustration on the part of the caregivers may also precipitate catastrophic reactions, as may accidents, or tasks that are too complicated for the person to complete.

Catastrophic reactions reflect the underlying tension and frustration of the disease. Because motor power is preserved until late in the course of Alzheimer's, these reactions can be quite frightening, destructive and dangerous.

Mood Disturbances

Mood changes are commonly seen in people with Alzheimer's disease. Our feelings are very much affected by the way we are able to think, and not only the damage to specific areas of the brain, but also the chilling realization of that damage, and the natural course of the disease, have three common effects on the emotional state of people with Alzheimer's.

Depression. This occurs in up to half the people with Alzheimer's disease, and it consists of withdrawal, despair, tearfulness and loss of the pleasures in life. These feelings of sadness are usually associated with a deterioration in sleep patterns, fatigue and changes in weight.

Diagnosing depression

Depression is common in older adults and very common in people who suffer from Alzheimer's disease. In one study almost 50 percent of those who had Alzheimer's suffered from depression. It is important to recognize depression because treatment can significantly improve the person's quality of life. To identify depression, look for these symptoms:

- persisting sadness and loss of interest in the pleasures of life
- withdrawal from social contacts
- weight change, insomnia, loss of appetite and energy
- feelings of worthlessness
- thoughts of death and suicide

The presence of depression can make Alzheimer's disease much worse, as depression causes a slowing down of thought processes and a clouding of insight and perception. Depression makes the ability to concentrate much poorer, so that learning suffers and memory fails. Most depression responds well to oral medicines, however, and treating it greatly improves the quality of life.

Anxiety. Excessive anxiety is also commonly seen in Alzheimer's disease, particularly in the earlier stages. Part of this anxiety results from simple and evident frustration at not being able to do basic tasks such as remembering the name of a neighbor, or organizing personal finances, or finding one's way back from the community park. Sometimes the anxieties result from the constant feeling of being disconnected—lost— in new surroundings, or from the delusions that are common early in the disease. People are often irritable, easily upset. They feel rushed and fluttery, as if they are not in control, and they worry constantly, often using such phrases as "I don't know what's going to happen" ... "I am so upset" ... "I hope it'll be all right."

Apathy. Withdrawal is common in Alzheimer's, and is often present fairly early in the disease, probably as a result of damage to the frontal lobe (the seat of insight, motivation and perception). These people don't seem too upset by their obvious mental deficiencies. They just shrug as if they don't care, and instead of reacting with concern and alarm, they appear uninterested in their loss of memory, their errors and confusion. They may say, "I'm too old for that sort of thing," or "Now, why would I be interested in that at my age?" They often progressively withdraw from encounters with their friends and family and appear emotionally blunted, indifferent both to their own state and increasing disability and to the world around them. This type of change in mood can be very demanding for caregivers, as the normal emotional response between loved ones is damaged by this cold detachment. Love becomes a one-way flow, and the caregiver feels used and hurt.

FOUR

Diagnosing Alzheimer's Disease

Alzheimer's disease can be diagnosed with absolute certainty only after death, when brain tissue can be examined microscopically to confirm the changes that are characteristic of the disease.

However, 90 percent of the time, a physician experienced in the field of dementia can make the diagnosis accurately through a combination of neurological examination and laboratory testing before death occurs. Alzheimer's disease is a progressive disorder, and as with many such disorders the diagnosis becomes more evident as time passes and more signs and symptoms develop. Thus, it may be quite difficult to diagnose Alzheimer's with certainty in its very early stages—where memory loss is the main problem—but diagnosis becomes much easier as time passes and other cognitive changes (such as difficulty with language, confusion and disorientation, problems with reasoning and calculation and so on) become evident.

The nose knows

The sensation of smell is carried by the olfactory nerve from the nose to the midbrain, where it is appreciated. The sense of smell is diminished in Alzheimer's and this loss worsens as the disease progresses. The midbrain shows damage early in Alzheimer's and this accounts for the loss of sense of smell. At first, people cannot discriminate among different smells. Eventually, they lose the sense of smell entirely. Some researchers believe that toxins or infections that could cause Alzheimer's may enter the brain through this port. According to this theory, the olfactory nerve acts as a conduit, taking these substances directly to the brain. In a similar manner, medicines to treat the disease may some day be transported directly to the brain via the nose.

A History Is Critical

When someone is brought to the doctor with memory loss and poor mental functioning, the doctor's first step is to take a careful history of the problem. This includes what exactly is wrong, how long it has been a problem and how it affects the person and those around him. Details of past illnesses, injuries and family history are also important. Most frequently, information from a family member (or friends) is crucial, because many people with early Alzheimer's disease have significant memory loss and poor insight and judgment. Interviewing the person usually gives limited information, so an accompanying member of the family can add important details. During this vital interview the "head turning" sign may be seen—when the person cannot recall a detail or answer, he or she turns to a family member for help.

All the signs and symptoms of Alzheimer's disease can be caused by a wide variety of drugs, so a careful history of drug use (both prescribed and over-the-counter medicines) is essential, with particular emphasis on sedative and tranquilizing drugs as well as sleeping pills. The details of alcohol use, education and job experience, exposure to toxic chemicals, psychiatric history (especially depression) and any recent change in emotional status or life stresses are all significant pieces of information elicited at this time.

The Physical Exam

After the history is taken, the person usually has a complete physical examination to rule out other diseases being the cause of the problem. Special focus is given to the neurological examination. Though there are no specific diagnostic neurological signs in Alzheimer's disease, rigid movement, a stooped posture and subtle changes in reflexes may be clues.

The doctor will pay careful attention to the ears and the eyes. Both poor hearing and vision commonly produce, or worsen, confusion, disorientation, inattention and poor mental

Jumping to conclusions

Martha had spent her life as a librarian in the school system, sharing with children the excitement of reading and the adventures of the printed page. When she retired, she withdrew into herself and her little house. She'd always worn glasses and had endured years of good-hearted kidding from her young students because the lenses in her glasses had become so thick. When her neighbors noted that she rarely left home they made a special effort to take her out frequently, but they were often discouraged by the condition of her house—it was filthy. Grime covered the walls, grease stained the counters and there was dirt everywhere. They felt certain that their beloved librarian was becoming "senile." They were quite surprised when the doctor did not confirm their diagnosis, but instead arranged for eye surgery to remove the dense cataracts that had worsened the borderline vision that she'd had for most of her life. The neighbors couldn't believe the change in Martha after the surgery, when she could see again. She was much happier, she was able to get about and do her yard work and shopping and she saw, for the first time in years, how squalid her house had become. The neighbors helped her clean her small house of the years of dust and grime. Her "senility" was gone.

Standardized Mini-Mental State Examination (SMMSE)

I am going to ask you some questions and give you some problems to solve. Please try to answer as best you can.

Maximum score

1. *(Allow 10 seconds for each reply.)*
   a) What year is this?   1
      (Accept exact answer only.)
   b) What season is this?   1
      (During last week of the old season or first week of a new season, accept either season.)
   c) What month of the year is this?   1
      (On the first day of new month, or last day of the previous month, accept either.)
   d) What is today's date?   1
      (Accept previous or next date; e.g., on the 7th accept the 6th or 8th.)
   e) What day of the week is this?   1
      (Accept exact answer only.)

2. *(Allow 10 seconds for each reply.)*
   a) What country are we in?   1
   b) What province/state/county are we in?   1
      (Accept exact answer only.)
   c) What city/town are we in?   1
      (Accept exact answer only.)
   d) *(In clinic)* What is the name of this hospital/building?   1
      (Accept exact name of hospital or institution only.)
      (In home) What is the street address of this house?   1
      (Accept exact answer only.)
   e) What floor are we on?   1

3. I am going to name 3 objects. After I have said all 3 names, I want you to repeat them. Remember what they are, because I am going to ask you to name them again in a few minutes.

   (Say them slowly at approximately one-second intervals.)

   Ball   Car   Man

   For repeated use:

   Bell   Jar   Fan
   Bill   Tar   Can
   Bull   War   Pan

   Please repeat the 3 items for me.   3

(Score 1 point for each correct reply on the first attempt. Allow 20 seconds for reply if subject did not repeat all 3; repeat until they are learned or up to a maximum of 5 times.)

4. Spell the word WORLD.   5
   (You may help the subject to spell the word correctly.)

   Now spell it backward please. *(Allow 30 seconds to spell it backward. If the subject cannot spell "world" even with assistance score 0.)*

5. Now, what were the 3 objects that I asked you to remember? 3

   Ball   Car   Man

   (Score 1 point for each correct response regardless of order; allow 10 seconds.)

6. Show wristwatch. Ask, "What is this called?"   1

   (Score 1 point for correct response. Accept "wristwatch" or "watch." Do not accept "clock," "time," etc. Allow 10 seconds.)

7. Show pencil. Ask, "What is this called?"   1

   (Score 1 point for correct response. Accept pencil only; score 0 for pen.)

8. I'd like you to repeat a phrase after me: "No ifs, ands or buts." 1

   (Allow 10 seconds for response. Score 1 point for a correct repetition. Must be exact; e.g., "no ifs or buts"—score 0.)

9. Say, "Read the words on this page and then do what it says."   1
   Hand subject a sheet with CLOSE YOUR EYES on it.

   (If subject just reads and does not then close eyes, you may repeat, "Read the words on this page and then do what it says," to a maximum of 3 times. Allow 10 seconds; score 1 point only if subject closes eyes. Subject does not have to read aloud.)

10. Ask if the subject is right-handed or left-handed.   3

    (Take a piece of paper, hold it up in front of subject and say, "Take this paper in your right/left hand [say "left" if right-handed and vice-versa], fold the paper in half once with both hands and put the paper down on the floor.")

    Takes paper in correct hand
    Folds it in half
    Puts it on the floor

    (Allow 30 seconds. Score 1 point for each instruction correctly executed.)

(continued)

11. Hand subject a pencil and paper.   I

Say, "Write any complete sentence on that piece of paper."

(Allow 30 seconds. Score 1 point. The sentence should make sense. Ignore spelling errors.)

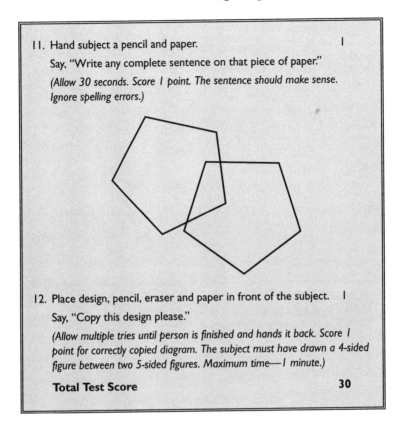

12. Place design, pencil, eraser and paper in front of the subject.   I

Say, "Copy this design please."

(Allow multiple tries until person is finished and hands it back. Score 1 point for correctly copied diagram. The subject must have drawn a 4-sided figure between two 5-sided figures. Maximum time—1 minute.)

Total Test Score   **30**

functioning in seniors. The sense of smell is usually markedly decreased or absent in Alzheimer's disease, but this is common in the elderly from other causes and is not diagnostic.

Assessing Brain Function

The next step in the diagnostic process is the most important one—assessing, by means of psychological testing, the functioning of the brain. The person is asked to complete, with the examiner's help, a series of simple questions and tasks carefully designed to show problems in thinking, reasoning and calculating. The commonest test used for this purpose is the Standardized Mini-Mental State Examination (SMMSE). It is worth reading to see how markedly abnormal the responses of people with Alzheimer's disease can be. (Note, too, the materials needed.) Most seniors have no trouble achieving a perfect score, and indeed scores between 26 and 30 are considered normal. Scores between 18 and 26 show mild but significant cognitive impairment and scores below this show moderate to severe loss of reasoning ability.

Additional psychological testing may be done to diagnose depression or other psychiatric problems, as symptoms of these disorders may mimic those of Alzheimer's disease.

Blood testing done in the diagnosis of Alzheimer's disease

Test	Reasons
Complete blood count	Anemia may cause many of the symptoms of dementia.
B_{12} and folic acid	A deficiency in vitamin B_{12} may cause dementia.
Blood sugar	Diabetes may cause dementia through blood sugar being too high or too low.
Kidney function	Kidney failure may cause clouding of mental functioning.
HIV and VDRL (syphilis)	These infections can cause dementia.
Thyroid hormone	High or low thyroid produces mental impairment.
Electrolytes	Imbalances may cause symptoms of dementia.
Calcium	Abnormalities may impair brain function.
Liver function	Dysfunction may cause symptoms of dementia.

Depending on individual cases, other blood tests may be ordered.

Laboratory Testing

Testing blood in the laboratory is also part of the diagnostic process, but because there are no specific blood tests or markers for Alzheimer's disease, this is done mainly to rule out other causes for the impaired mental functioning and memory loss.

Imaging Techniques

Ideally, to diagnose Alzheimer's disease, doctors like to get a good look at the brain itself, and this is the next step in the process: trying to obtain a graphic representation of the neuron loss and other changes that characterize the disease. There are three different techniques.

CT or CAT scan (computerized axial tomography). The patient lies inside a large, hollow tube containing an X-ray machine that takes pictures of "slices" of the brain in sequence. These add up to a three-dimensional image of the inside of the brain. Often, CT scans in Alzheimer's disease show atrophy, or shrinkage, of the brain. However, the brains of many seniors atrophy as they become older, so the process of brain-cell loss is not diagnostic. Some CT scan techniques are so accurate that they can diagnose Alzheimer's disease with a high degree of probability by examining the loss of volume in specific parts of the brain (such as the hippocampus, the seat of short-term memory). CT scans are also useful in the diagnostic process because they rule out other causes of abnormal mental function—multiple small strokes, brain tumors or hydrocephalus, for example.

MRI (magnetic resonance imaging). This form of brain imaging does not involve X-rays. Instead, it measures the tiny energy charges when human tissue is briefly exposed to a strong magnetic field. It produces a much more detailed analysis of brain structures than the CT scan does. It often picks up smaller anatomical changes (such as multiple minor strokes).

Cause of death

The average duration of the disease from diagnosis to death is eight to nine years. The progress of the disease varies somewhat from person to person, but ultimately it damages brain tissue, leading to progressive weakness and immobility. The consequences of this increasing debility, not the primary brain damage, eventually kill those with the disease. In the final states, people lose the ability to walk and swallow. Once they can't walk they become bedridden and run the risk of developing blood clots, pressure sores and infections. Inability to swallow leads to malnutrition and pneumonia from inhaling food into the lungs. The majority succumb to pneumonia—"the old man's friend," blood clots to the lungs, complications from urinary tract infections, or pressure sores.

SPECT (single photon emission computed tomography) or *PET (positron emission tomography)*. Both CT and MRI scans show structural change only—the loss of neurons seen in Alzheimer's disease—but SPECT or PET scans can actually test for a change in the function of brain tissue. When brain cells are damaged they use less glucose. The patient is given an injection of glucose (sugar solution) with a radioactive "tracer" and the glucose circulates to the brain. These two imaging techniques measure the use of the glucose in various areas of the brain. In Alzheimer's disease there is decreased use of glucose over the frontal and temporal lobes.

FIVE

Reactions: Denial, Anger and Depression

It's hard to accept a diagnosis of Alzheimer's. It can seem so harsh and unfair. When people first hear that they or a loved one has the disease, they usually go through four stages—denial, anger, depression and bargaining—before they finally come to acceptance. It is normal to pass through these four stages, and it is not uncommon to have feelings of denial, anger, sadness and even some acceptance all at once. It is important to recognize these feelings and accept them as natural, but it is also important to let go of the denial, anger and depression, because they harm everyone concerned. These emotions waste energy and diminish the ability to manage difficult tasks such as communicating, helping, caring and understanding. People who are depressed or angry are preoccupied, distracted, unable to focus on the task at hand. Angry people take their anger out on themselves and those around them.

"I Want to Know for Sure"

Mrs. Kent visited the doctor with her daughter, Susan, and her husband. Susan had phoned beforehand to say that her mother had taken Mr. Kent to three different specialists, who had all told her he had Alzheimer's disease. Once they mentioned Alzheimer's, Mrs. Kent never went back to see them. She became angry when anyone tried to make her accept reality.

The problem is that we cannot diagnose Alzheimer's with 100 percent certainty without a brain biopsy. A brain biopsy is very invasive: it requires drilling through the skull and removing a piece of brain tissue. If the biopsy of brain tissue shows the unmistakable physical changes of Alzheimer's, the condition is called "definite" Alzheimer's. But the biopsy does not change the treatment, so we don't perform the biopsy. The family doctor and specialists investigated Mr. Kent's memory loss with blood tests and CT scans of the brain and diagnosed the cause of the memory loss as "probable" Alzheimer's.

Although a diagnosis without a biopsy is called "probable," it is about 90 percent certain. But Mrs. Kent heard "probable" and became stuck on this single word. She wanted a definite answer, and "probable" suggested to her that the doctors were only guessing. She focused on the uncertainty and blocked everything else out. When her family doctor refused to send her to yet another specialist, she changed family doctors and got appointments with different specialists. She was going round and round in circles. She would not allow home-care workers into the house, yet she phoned Susan every day complaining that she was exhausted and that Susan was not helping enough.

Poor Mr. Kent was not getting any help. He was living with a very angry woman who blamed him for everything. Not surprisingly, he was a handful. In the doctor's office he was agitated. He kept walking out of the room looking for his wife. When she was with him, he kept pulling at her and badgering her to go home. He had a very short attention span and could not sit down to talk, look at a book or relax. He was constantly on the go. He demanded one-on-one attention all the time. He was getting up at night and wandering out of the house, so his wife could not sleep for fear that he would leave. He was sleeping during the day when she was doing the housework. She was exhausted, burned out, alone and isolated.

When the assessment was finished, the doctor sat down with Mrs. Kent and asked her how many other doctors she had been to see, and she glared. "A few." He asked her what they had told her and she replied, "They don't know what the problem is. They told me they weren't sure what he had." Then he asked her what they thought her husband had and she replied, "None of them would say for sure if it was Alzheimer's. They only said it might be."

The doctor told her he was certain Mr. Kent had Alzheimer's disease. She became angry and burst out, "Yes, but can you say for sure?" He replied, "Yes, he has Alzheimer's. I am certain." She became even more angry. "Are you absolutely sure—can you say this with 100 percent certainty?" He answered honestly, "No. Nobody can. You can choose to go to more doctors and hear the same thing again and again, or you can listen to what I have to tell you and try to accept it. If you don't listen and accept help, you are going to get very ill and you will not be able to help your husband anymore. You will drive your family away and your husband will have to go to a nursing home sooner than he should. You keep hoping for a cure. Well, I can tell you now with 100 percent certainty that there is no cure. You are in denial. You are angry. You have to let go of your anger. You have to come to terms with this disease or it will kill you both. Your anger is destroying your life. If you want help, I will help you. If not, walk out that door right now. It's up to you. I can help you if you let me. Otherwise you will remain where you are, alone, isolated, suffering, stuck like a car spinning its wheels in mud."

Mrs. Kent stood up to go. Denial is like a wall. You have to hammer away at it by repeating the same thing over and over. Eventually you break it down. The doctor knew he was going to get just one more shot at it. He changed his tone and held out his hands to her.

"Mrs. Kent, please listen to me. I do this for a living day after day. I've seen over five thousand people with this disease, and their families. This denial is damaging you, your husband and your daughter. Unless you come out of denial and let go of the anger and depression, no one can help you. When people try to help, you push them away.

"You want someone to tell you your husband doesn't have Alzheimer's. But it's not going to happen. You're angry at me because I'm telling you the same thing as every other doctor. You're afraid of the diagnosis and you'll do anything to avoid

---

Diagnosing Alzheimer's

Physicians have devised a classification system for the diagnosis of Alzheimer's disease, based on relative degrees of certainty.

Definite Alzheimer's disease	Microscopic evidence of the characteristic brain changes at the time of autopsy in someone with typical signs and symptoms.
Probable Alzheimer's disease	The commonest diagnosis during life. It can be made with confidence in someone who has a typical onset and slow progression of mental disability, with no other systemic brain disease that would cause the memory loss and other cognitive changes.
Possible Alzheimer's disease	The diagnosis often suggested for someone who is early in the course of the disease, before all the typical features have been observed, but in whom no other cause or disease process is found to explain the difficulties in memory and decreased mental function.

This classification system is very accurate—in one study 90 percent of those diagnosed as having "probable" Alzheimer's disease were confirmed at autopsy with diagnostic pathological changes.

it. But there is no avoiding it. Give up now. Let's face it together. If you allow me, I will help you. But you have to listen to me. I'll be your coach if you let me. Don't blame yourself. Don't blame your husband. Let's try to help him. He needs our help."

Mrs. Kent wavered at the door, not knowing whether to stay or go. Finally she slumped back in the chair. She started crying, but the doctor had finally gotten through to her. After the tears, they talked for a long time and she came to see him regularly after that.

Dealing with Anger and Depression

Anger is a very dangerous emotion. It is powerful and hard to control. Angry people are hard to be around. They are exhausting. Anger creates anger, yet the worst thing you can do with an angry person is to become angry back at them. When someone is angry, just let the outburst go by. Don't react until the anger has burned itself out. Then it is possible to step in to help.

Depression can manifest itself in many ways: sleep disturbance, loss of appetite, weight gain, loss of energy, loss of interest, anxiety, self-neglect, even suicide. The good news is that there are many effective ways to deal with depression. But depression can also lead to anger, and there is no drug for that. It takes control, patience and time to work through anger. First it's important to recognize it, in ourselves and others. Then it's important to let the feelings go. The anger and depression that come with a diagnosis of Alzheimer's are normal but debilitating. It takes time to get over them, to eventually accept the disease. Treatment of anger and depression are discussed further in chapter 9.

If you yourself have Alzheimer's, you may find it helpful to take stock of how well you are doing. Are you in denial, angry, depressed, or have you accepted the disease? Are you coping, or are you stressed out? Before you can learn to cope with the

Elder abuse

People with Alzheimer's are probably more vulnerable to abuse than any other group in society. About 4 percent of older adults living in the community are abused by a family member, friend or caregiver. Older adults are at increased risk if they have poor family relationships, or if caregivers are substance abusers, have emotional or psychiatric problems or are burned out trying to provide care. Abusers are usually dependent on the older adult and the older adult is dependent on them. This is co-dependency. The abuse may not be intentional. Abuse usually gets worse over time. One of the greatest problems is that since older adults are dependent on or related to their abusers, they often feel responsible, afraid or ashamed to report the behavior.

Signs of abuse:
- The older adult may be depressed, anxious or afraid of the abuser.
- His or her behavior changes when the abuser is present.
- The older adult may not speak for himself or herself and may refer everything to the abuser.
- The caregiver may be aggressive or insulting, or talk for the older adult.
- The abuser may even show excessive concern for the older adult.
- Appointments are missed.
- Money disappears.
- There are delays in seeking treatment or care.
- The older person has unexplained bruises or scratches.
- The older adult has a standard of living that is below what he/she can afford, and food, clothing or living conditions are inadequate.
- The caregiver deliberately isolates or separates the older adult from other family or friends, or may not want to leave the older person alone with others.

If you suspect that someone close to you is being abused, listen to the person and try to interview him or her apart from the suspected abuser. It is important not to confront the abuser. Try to understand the relationship and why it is abusive. Don't blame the abuser; provide support. The abuser often provides a great deal of support to the older adult and it is important to increase support to both. Get help from professional caregivers, family, friends, physicians or clergy. The first step is to gain the trust of the abuser and the person being abused. Often it is not possible to separate them because they need each other. In most cases, the best we can do is provide support to both. Abuse is a complex and difficult situation that is frequently chronic and hard to unravel.

disease, you must accept it, set your goals, educate yourself and develop your care plan. If you are a caregiver you are probably feeling a lot of uncertainty and stress.

It's Not Only the Patient Who Suffers

If you are caring for someone with Alzheimer's, the disease is affecting you too. The entire family suffers from the effects of Alzheimer's disease. Answer the questions in the box below and see how much it is affecting your life. With this as a baseline you will see more clearly what problems you have. Until you know what your problems are, you can't start to solve them. Remember that it's impossible to care for someone with Alzheimer's if you don't care for yourself first and foremost. It's not selfish—it's survival. If you don't take care of yourself, the disease will kill both of you.

When you answer the 15 questions honestly, you will have insight into how this disease has changed your life. The higher you score, the greater your stress level. Caregivers often feel angry, frustrated, depressed and, above all, trapped. They feel inadequate—they feel they are not doing enough, caring enough, loving enough. The pressing needs are like a bottomless pit. Their "golden" years become a nightmare, as they watch a loved one disintegrate before their eyes. They wonder how God could be so cruel, and ask, "What did I do to deserve this?" Don't worry if you feel like this—it's completely normal. If you feel like walking out the door and never coming back, that's normal too. You need to share these feelings with family, friends, your doctor or an Alzheimer's support group. First, recognize the feelings. Next, talk them out with people who understand and can offer a sympathetic ear. Start by working on the easier aspects, until you can let go of your negative feelings; then progress through the more difficult feelings, until you can let go of them and start living again.

Caregivers: do you have these feelings?

	Yes	No
1. The person demands more help than he/she needs.	[ ]	[ ]
2. You spend too much time caring for the person.	[ ]	[ ]
3. He/she makes you feel angry/resentful.	[ ]	[ ]
4. He/she makes you feel sad/depressed.	[ ]	[ ]
5. He/she makes you feel embarrassed/anxious.	[ ]	[ ]
6. You are uncertain about your future (for you and the person).	[ ]	[ ]
7. You are afraid you will not be able to afford care for the person.	[ ]	[ ]
8. You are afraid you will not be able to manage in the future.	[ ] [ ]	[ ] [ ]
9. Caring for him/her has made you ill.	[ ]	[ ]
10. Caring for him/her has damaged your social life.	[ ]	[ ]
11. Caring for him/her has taken all your money.	[ ]	[ ]
12. Caring for him/her has taken your freedom.	[ ]	[ ]
13. Caring for him/her has taken your privacy.	[ ]	[ ]
14. Caring for him/her has taken control of your life.	[ ]	[ ]
15. You have failed to provide proper care for him/her.	[ ]	[ ]

Alzheimer's is a journey—at times painful, at times sad, at times funny and always challenging. It challenges us all to consider the purpose and meaning of our lives. It brings out our most human qualities—love, compassion and understanding. Few of us who go on the journey finish it the way we started. It changes us forever. It has so much to teach us about the futility of so many values that we previously held high. Alzheimer's has no respect for money, power, position or achievement. It creates victims and survivors. But by understanding the disease—and your role as a caregiver—you can keep yourself from becoming an additional victim of the disease.

SIX

Caring for Someone with Alzheimer's Disease

People have heard so many horror stories about Alzheimer's that they say, "As long as it's not Alzheimer's, I don't mind. I can take anything but that." They believe that everyone who gets the disease loses dignity and becomes violent and unmanageable. Families who come to terms with the disease can handle it well, preserve the person's dignity and minimize suffering.

We cannot avoid suffering. Sometimes the best we can do is accept it and support one another through it. Caregivers must learn how to develop a care plan and how to care. One of the biggest problems faced by those who have the disease and their caregivers is deciding where to start. The disease can seem so overwhelming at first.

What follows is a four-point plan. It won't solve all the problems, but it can make life a lot easier for everyone. Start at the beginning and follow the steps laid out. Take one step at a time. Don't try to do everything at once.

Should you tell people they have Alzheimer's disease?

In an effort to protect their loved ones, family members often wonder if the diagnosis of Alzheimer's should be withheld from the person involved. By not telling the person, they hope to spare him or her the full anguish of the disease, and they feel that not mentioning the diagnosis will be emotionally easier for everyone. Sometimes the person has specifically asked not to be told. However, many groups, including Alzheimer's societies, strongly recommend telling the truth, and emphasize that we all have the right to know what is happening to our minds and our bodies. Not telling the person undermines the trust that is essential to adequate care.

An actual diagnosis explains what most sufferers already recognize as abnormal thinking and behavior, and this allows them the dignity of at least understanding their decline.

Telling the person enables him or her to participate in decisions about long-term care, including living wills, placement in nursing homes, medication trials and so on. In addition, day-to-day decisions such as when to stop driving and how to make the most of the remaining good times can be reached by the family together. All in all, people with Alzheimer's have the right to know their diagnosis, even though it is painful to tell them.

There are four questions to ask yourself. Each will be covered in greater detail in the sections that follow.

1. Is this Alzheimer's?
2. At what stage is the disease?
3. What's the overall care plan?
4. How will you manage day-to-day problems?

Is This Alzheimer's?

Alzheimer's causes short-term memory loss. If there is no memory loss, it's not Alzheimer's. Refer back to the explanation of short-term memory in chapter 3 and diagnosing Alzheimer's in chapter 4. Establish the diagnosis before proceeding. Rule out other causes of memory loss, and treat depression if it is present.

At What Stage Is the Disease?

Alzheimer's is the most common progressive dementia. It follows a steady, predictable but individual path. It is important to determine, as accurately as possible, where the person is along this path. This will help you to understand why he or she is acting a certain way. Just as important, you will be able to predict how the disease will progress. You will be able to follow a plan that lays out what to do at the different stages of the disease, and it will help you develop a personalized care program for the person's changing needs.

The course of the disease may seem random, but it's not. The easy-to-read FAST (Functional Assessment Staging) scale, developed by Dr. Barry Reisberg, describes seven distinct phases. This simple map lays out the disease and marks the seven steps on the journey that caregivers and the person with Alzheimer's will take. The disease nearly always follows this course, so if you are prepared, there will be few surprises. When you plan, you begin to deal with the problems you will face even before they happen.

What's the Overall Care Plan?

Each stage of the disease has different challenges. To meet these, it is necessary to have an overall strategy for managing each stage. As the disease progresses, the problems change and new issues arise. Caregivers face a fresh set of problems at each turn in the road. If you have a care map, you can deal with the challenges you face now and plan for those that lie ahead. This ensures that you will provide the best care possible. You can keep the person safe and comfortable, and guarantee the best quality of life possible in spite of this devastating disease.

Here are some practical guidelines to assist you at each stage. Again, it is important not only to deal with the problems at hand but also to plan for the next stage. For example,

Stages in Alzheimer's disease (A.D.)

(Adapted from the FAST)

FAST stage	Characteristics	Clinical diagnosis	Estimated duration*
1	Normal	Normal adult	
2	Subjective problems finding the right word. Forgetting familiar names or where one has placed familiar objects. No problem in employment or social situations.	Normal aged adult. This is also known as "benign forgetful-ness." SMMSE score 27 to 30†	
3 A.D. starts here	Problems at work (poor perfor-mance). Problems in word and name finding become obvious to family. Person gets lost traveling to familiar locations. Poor concentration. Memory prob-lems obvious in conversation. Person repeats self and loses track. Difficulty learning new information.	Early Alzheimer's SMMSE score about 23 to 26	7 years
4	Problems with concentration; forgets current events. Memory problems start to interfere with social behavior. Requires assistance handling finances, planning a dinner party.	Mild Alzheimer's disease SMMSE score about 18 to 22	2 years
5	Requires assistance with basic activities of daily living such as grooming and dressing; is unable to remember significant facts such as grandchildren's names. Is disoriented about time or place. Can't understand or carry out complex tasks such as following a recipe or shopping.	Moderate Alzheimer's disease SMMSE score about 12 to 17	18 months
6	Requires assistance dressing, bathing, toileting, even eating. Is unaware of recent events in life; may forget name of spouse. Sleep disturbance; up at night.	Late Alzheimer's disease SMMSE score about 5, range 3 to 10.	30 months

	Personality and emotional changes with anxiety, delusions and agitation or aggression. Loses bladder control.		
7	Speech limited to about a half-dozen words; eventually this progresses to complete loss. Can't walk, sit up, smile or swallow. Loses bowel control.	Severe Alzheimer's disease	up to 6 years

*In those who survive and progress to the subsequent deterioration stage
†Standardized Mini-Mental State Examination; see chapter 4

if the person is mentally competent in stage three but will become incompetent in stage four, get any legal documents signed in stage three; if you wait too long, it will be too late.

Stages 1 and 2. Normal Aging

Although we do not know what causes Alzheimer's, we can offer some good advice about reducing the risk of memory loss. Stay healthy, keep active, eat a balanced diet (low fat and low salt) with lots of fruits and vegetables. Have your blood pressure checked regularly. Get to your ideal weight. Use your brain—reading, doing crossword puzzles—and stay involved. Better to wear out than to rust out! If you are over 55, talk to your doctor about taking enteric-coated ASA (aspirin) each day, with your main meal. Take vitamin E according to your doctor's recommendation. Women should take estrogen after menopause unless there is a strong history of breast cancer; ask your doctor for advice here too. Avoid excessive alcohol, and avoid head injuries. Stay positive and optimistic.

Stage 3. Early Alzheimer's

Once Alzheimer's is diagnosed after a careful, comprehensive

Care plan for person living with caregiver

FAST stage		Estimated duration
1		
2	Will	
	Powers of attorney (financial and personal care)	
	Advance health care directive (living will)	
	Use of dosette for medication	
	Calendar reminder for appointments (kept by phone)	
3 A.D. starts here	Education of patient and family by Alzheimer's society	7 years
	Family member accompanies to appointments	
	Family fills the dosette and supervises medication	
	Check safety in the home (kettle, burners, cooking)	
	Churches and clubs to help	
	Check driving, finances, shopping	
	Start cholinesterase inhibitor (e.g., donepezil, rivastigmine, galantamine)	
	Consider starting vitamin E	
	Consider starting enteric-coated ASA (aspirin)	
4	Discuss how much support family/spouse provide	2 years
	Home-care programs	
	Day programs	
	Day care	
	Papers for placement in nursing home completed	
	In-home respite care and friendly visitors	
	Consider respite care (during stages 4 and 5)	
	Wandering Person Registry	
5	Caregiver support	18 months
	Short-stay respite care in a facility	
6	Nursing-home care; need secure unit if wandering	30 months
	Support caregiver in restarting life alone	
7	Secure unit	up to 6 years
	Grief and bereavement counseling for family	

Care plan for person living alone

FAST stage		Estimated duration
I		
2	Will Powers of attorney Advance health care directive Use of dosette for medication Calendar reminder for appointments, diary and so on	
3 A.D. starts here	Test driving Use calendar and message book Pharmacy to fill dosette. Start cholinesterase inhibitor (e.g., donepezil, rivastigmine, galantamine) Banks to pay bills Consider moving to seniors' apartment or retirement home Education regarding Alzheimer's disease. Discuss what you would want if your memory/function and so on deteriorates. Revise/update advance health care directive. Join Alzheimer's society, friendly visitor, and investigate/ start a day program Check finances, cooking, medication, shopping and so on Family member accompanies to doctors' appointments	7 years
4	Home-care supports (including social work for family) Consider moving in with family member(s) Likely transfer to care facility at this stage Wandering Person Registry	2 years
5	Most people who live alone will be in an institution by now Make a biography for the care facility	18 months
6	Nursing-home care	30 months
7	Grief and bereavement counseling for family	up to 6 years

assessment, join an Alzheimer's society for education and support. This is also the time for the person with Alzheimer's to get legal and financial affairs in order. He or she will need a will, an advance health care directive (living will) and power of attorney for property and personal care.

Safety issues are important at this stage. If the person is still driving, take precautions. Travel with the person and observe how he or she drives. Does he or she get lost, lose concentration, forget proper signals and exceed speed limits? If there are concerns, advise the doctor, who will order either a regular driving test or a tailored driving test in a center that specializes in testing people with Alzheimer's.

If the person is responsible for taking his or her own medications, at this stage count doses and check if some are skipped or too many are taken. A dosette—a segmented pill box with a compartment for each day of the week—is often useful. It will enable you to count out the pills and determine how regularly they are being taken.

At this stage, the person is at risk of financial abuse by con artists. People with Alzheimer's disease have difficulty keeping track of things, and will forget to pay bills or will pay the same bill over and over. The purpose of obtaining power of attorney is not to take over the person's affairs but to supervise, to make sure finances are handled properly. For example, bills

Driving and Alzheimer's

In the twentieth century, the automobile has become the symbol of freedom. Taking away a driving license from a senior is an enormous blow to independence and self-esteem. In the early stages it may still be possible to drive safely, but eventually everyone with Alzheimer's loses this ability. The warning signs that the person is becoming unsafe include inattention, slow reaction time and poor driving judgment—for example, the person drives through stop signs, changes lanes without checking or signaling, misses red lights and responds slowly or inappropriately to hazards and dangerous situations. If you have a concern, it is important to err on the side of safety and tell your family doctor. He or she will evaluate the person and arrange a driving test.

can be paid automatically through the bank. Allow the person to handle as much as possible. Don't take over for the sake of taking over. Keep the person involved.

When someone with Alzheimer's is living alone, his or her family may become concerned about nutrition. How well is the fridge stocked and how good are the person's cooking abilities? Assist with shopping and try to get the person to use a microwave to heat up prepared meals, as conventional ovens are more dangerous. Stock up on easy-to-cook meals. Consider Meals on Wheels.

People at this early stage usually deny memory loss. They become upset when others try to tell them what to do, because they honestly believe that the problem is being exaggerated. Resentment increases as caregivers start to intrude into their lives. If possible, try to get the person to talk to the doctor with you about long-term plans. Ask whom he or she wants to manage health and personal affairs, and money and property. Find out now how the person feels about living in an institution, and when he or she would agree to go there. This may be a very difficult conversation, but it will give both of you comfort eventually. At this stage you may both feel confused and frightened, even terrified at the prospect of what lies ahead. It's important to get on the right track early. It will make matters easier all the way along.

The natural tendency is to try to carry on and pretend the disease does not exist. If you do this, not only do you lose a valuable opportunity to get these things done, but it will be a hundred times more difficult, if not impossible, when the memory loss gets worse. Later, when the person loses competency, he or she will be unable to sign papers to grant others power of attorney. This means the government will become involved, and the family will have to work through the courts to be appointed guardian to make decisions on the person's behalf. If you don't make arrangements at this stage, the problems just build up. Plan; don't wait for a crisis.

Stage 4. Mild Alzheimer's

At this stage people develop problems with the basic requirements of daily living such as dressing and hygiene. The emphasis shifts from planning to helping with daily activities. The best strategy is to lay out clothes and assist with bathing and grooming. At first, gently remind the person, "It's time to have a bath, I'll run it for you." Later, as the disease progresses, the person may put on clothes incorrectly, and you will have to lay out clothes in sequence. Try to provide help in an upbeat manner, and do your best to make tasks fun. If the person fails, don't correct unless it's necessary. Don't scold, but gently suggest, for example, "That vest looks better the other way around. Let's try it that way."

Up to this point most caregivers can manage alone. Now they start to feel overwhelmed. They are caring 24 hours a day, seven days a week. They have no time to themselves. Their relatives follow them around and are becoming increasingly dependent on them. Caregivers burn out at this stage if they seek help too late.

You Can't Do It Alone

The Canadian Alzheimer Society slogan is "You Can't Do It Alone"; the slogan of the American Alzheimer's Association is "Someone to Stand by You." Most caregivers come to understand the significance of these thoughts at this stage. Some wait too long to get or accept help and they burn out. Caregiver burnout is characterized by exhaustion, frustration and anger. Plan to accept help. You will need it.

There are a variety of ways to get it. Support workers can come into the home to help with personal care and household chores. Some workers spend time with the person with Alzheimer's to give the caregiver a break. In many areas, Alzheimer's society volunteers will take the person for a walk and give the caregiver additional free time. Talk to your doctor and your local Alzheimer's organization to find out what's available in your area. Even the best caregivers need help. You should not consider it a failure if you do. Caregiving is like playing a sport such as hockey. Hockey players don't stay on the ice for the whole game. They need to sit on the bench and take a break at times. Caregivers also need time out.

Another way to get a break at this stage is to enroll the person in a day-care center, to meet others and become involved in a range of activities. Often people with Alzheimer's refuse to go to day-care centers at first. If caregivers go along with them, they soon get used to it. Day programs are widely available and should become a part of the routine. As the disease progresses, people can go more often, because the caregivers will need more and more help as the work becomes heavier and more demanding.

It is also useful to have an occupational therapist come into the home to give valuable advice on how to make the home safe. A whole range of modifications can be made to keep the person safe and increase his or her function. These are discussed later in this chapter.

Stages 5 and 6. Moderate and Late Alzheimer's

At this stage, people require 24-hour care. They can't be left alone; they have to have constant supervision. They need to be washed, dressed and groomed, and may have to be fed and toileted. Some will not remember family members; some will get lost in their own homes. Others will want to go home to their parents, who have been dead for 20 years. If they are allowed to nap during the day, some will get up at night and ask for breakfast.

Many caregivers refuse to accept that the person will have to live in an institution. They try to hang on, and finally, when they burn out and can't continue, they are devastated that they must admit their loved one to a nursing home. They did not plan for the move and must now start looking about, filling out papers and trying to choose a home that is nearby and provides good-quality care. This is the worst time to do this; it should have been organized as part of your care plan.

Nursing-home care should be considered and discussed when the person starts to have trouble with the simple activities of daily living. People with Alzheimer's who are living alone may have to go to a care facility much sooner. It is important to plan ahead. Too many caregivers and families leave it to the last minute, and have to take the first place they can get.

When caregivers are asked if they have considered a nursing home, many reply, "Never. I will never let him/her go to a nursing home. I want to keep him/her at home." If this is the way you feel, ask yourself four questions:

- "What will happen if he/she does not recognize me anymore?"
- "What will happen if he/she is incontinent of urine and stool?"
- "What will happen if I have to lift him/her in and out of bed?"
- "Will I keep him/her at home then?"

This is harsh, but it has to be done. Statistics show that 90 percent of people with Alzheimer's will need facility care for some time in the advanced stage. Caregivers have to plan that the person *will* go to a nursing home. If you learn how to manage the disease and accept help, you will keep your loved one at home much longer. But eventually the vast majority of caregivers, whether they like it or not, cannot provide enough help. Most are relieved when those they are caring for are admitted to a nursing home in the end.

Caregivers, make arrangements ahead of time. A person should not be moved to a nursing home in a crisis or an emergency, if possible. The move should be planned. If the move occurs because the caregiver becomes ill and goes into the hospital, the rest of the family have to step in to manage the person with the disease. Then they have to cope with one person in hospital and the other at home, with little help.

How Will You Manage Day-to-Day Problems?

The biggest challenge for caregivers isn't seeing to the mundane tasks—washing, dressing, cooking, handling the finances. For most, it's managing the behavior changes over the course of the disease: the abnormal actions and personality changes. Different behavior problems occur at different stages.

Behavior is defined as any form of human expression; it is complex and highly individual. Damage to the brain cells can cause severe changes in behavior. In managing any behavior problem, there are three steps to follow.

First, describe the behavior and its possible causes. If the cause can be removed or modified, the behavior may get better or disappear. Decide whether you must act—if safety is compromised, for example—or whether you can ignore the behavior.

Second, learn coping strategies. Try different strategies to see what works and what doesn't, following a problem-solving, common-sense approach.

Third, assess the effect of your coping strategies. If one worked, use it again. If it didn't, don't give up. As long as it didn't make the behavior worse, you can try to go with the flow and remain as flexible as possible. It may work the next time. Review your successes and failures and try again. Seek help for behavior that you can't change.

Dysfunctional Behavior Rating Instrument (DBRI)

How often has the person had any of the following behaviors in the past few weeks, and how much of a problem has it been? Complete this checklist periodically to track behavior problems. High scores are indicators of caregiver stress.

Circle the number that best applies:	How often does this occur?	How much of a problem is this?
	0 Never	0 No problem
	1 About every two weeks	1 Very little problem
	2 About once a week	2 Little problem
	3 More than once a week	3 Somewhat of a problem
	4 At least once daily	4 Moderate problem
	5 More than five times a day	5 Great problem

1. Asked same questions over and over	0 1 2 3 4 5	0 1 2 3 4 5
2. Repeated stories over and over	0 1 2 3 4 5	0 1 2 3 4 5
3. Became angry	0 1 2 3 4 5	0 1 2 3 4 5
4. Was withdrawn (did not speak or do anything unless asked)	0 1 2 3 4 5	0 1 2 3 4 5
5. Was demanding	0 1 2 3 4 5	0 1 2 3 4 5
6. Was afraid to be left alone	0 1 2 3 4 5	0 1 2 3 4 5
7. Was aggressive	0 1 2 3 4 5	0 1 2 3 4 5
8. Was hiding things	0 1 2 3 4 5	0 1 2 3 4 5
9. Was suspicious	0 1 2 3 4 5	0 1 2 3 4 5
10. Had temper outbursts	0 1 2 3 4 5	0 1 2 3 4 5
11. Expressed delusions (thoughts) that:		
• spouse was "not my husband/wife"	0 1 2 3 4 5	0 1 2 3 4 5
• home was "not my home"	0 1 2 3 4 5	0 1 2 3 4 5
• there were "people in the house"	0 1 2 3 4 5	0 1 2 3 4 5
• "people were stealing things"	0 1 2 3 4 5	0 1 2 3 4 5
• other: _____	0 1 2 3 4 5	0 1 2 3 4 5
12. Had hallucinations:		
• saw things that were not there	0 1 2 3 4 5	0 1 2 3 4 5

• heard things or people that were not there	0 1 2 3 4 5	0 1 2 3 4 5
• other: _____	0 1 2 3 4 5	0 1 2 3 4 5
13. Was agitated, e.g., pacing	0 1 2 3 4 5	0 1 2 3 4 5
14. Was crying	0 1 2 3 4 5	0 1 2 3 4 5
15. Was frustrated	0 1 2 3 4 5	0 1 2 3 4 5
16. Wandered, got lost in house, on property or elsewhere	0 1 2 3 4 5	0 1 2 3 4 5
17. Was up at night	0 1 2 3 4 5	0 1 2 3 4 5
18. Wanted to leave	0 1 2 3 4 5	0 1 2 3 4 5
19. Kept changing mind	0 1 2 3 4 5	0 1 2 3 4 5
20. Refused to cooperate	0 1 2 3 4 5	0 1 2 3 4 5
21. Behaved embarrassingly in public	0 1 2 3 4 5	0 1 2 3 4 5
22. Had other behaviors not mentioned	0 1 2 3 4 5	0 1 2 3 4 5
_____		
_____		
_____		

There are some basic rules to follow in managing any behavior in Alzheimer's disease. Use the Dysfunctional Behavior Rating Instrument (DBRI) to measure how many different behaviors you are dealing with. The DBRI provides a checklist of behavior problems commonly found in people with Alzheimer's disease. On average, caregivers report ten or more of these in a week. The variety and frequency add to the challenge they face in coping with the person with Alzheimer's. Once you know the problems, you can learn how to manage them.

Describe the Action or Behavior

To understand the behavior, begin by describing what you see. Remember that someone may shout or pace because of anger, fear, worry, anxiety, depression or pain. Try not to "interpret" the behavior. Just describe what you see: shouting or pacing.

What Were the Causes or Triggers?

Were there any clues? Did you see or feel it coming? Is it likely related to a medical problem or a change in the person's environment? Is it worse in certain rooms, at a particular time of the day or with certain caregivers? For any behavior, there are common causes or triggers that make the behavior worse. Whenever a behavior gets worse, go through this checklist and try to relieve the causes or triggers.

Medical Causes

- new drugs, or changes in doses of old drugs
- disease other than Alzheimer's (viral infections, cystitis, arthritis)
- poor vision or hearing
- pain
- fever
- constipation or inability to pass urine (retention)

Environmental Causes

- hunger, thirst (which may be difficult for the person to explain)
- loss of sleep
- too much stimulation or stress in the environment
- not enough stimulation, boredom
- need for physical activity
- too many complicated demands or unfamiliar people or places
- too hot or too cold
- too dark, bright or noisy
- not enough supervision or communication

What Are the Effects on the Person?
What happens to the voice, actions, mood, appetite, emotions or energy? How is the person afterward? How does the behavior or action affect others?

What Are the Effects on You, the Caregiver?
How do you as caregiver respond to the behavior? Do you ignore it? Do you give more attention or do you punish the person for it? A caregiver's response will affect the way the behavior plays itself out. Make sure your responses are not making matters worse.

Guidelines for Managing Behavior Problems

Different behaviors have different causes and require different coping strategies. In managing any behavior, the caregiver must stay in control and remain calm. As a general rule, it doesn't help to try to reason with the person. It is usually more effective to try to distract the person. Behavior management principles may seem difficult, but they can be learned.

Remember that the person can't control these behaviors and is not responsible for them. He or she should not be punished. People with Alzheimer's disease do not learn from punishment. It's abusive to punish them. It will not help, and only makes matters worse.

Here are some guidelines for managing behavior problems in general. Specific strategies for particular behavior problems are given later in the chapter.

Learn Coping Strategies
• Consider what coping strategies have been tried and what effect they have had on the behavior.
• Keep a log of the behaviors, possible causes, patterns, triggers, actions taken and responses.

- Ignore bad behaviors as much as possible and reward good ones.
- Stand back and keep calm.
- Use your voice, touch, music and familiar objects or activities to distract the person and create a tranquil mood.
- Always reassure the person; say that you care and want to help.

Develop and Stick to Your Routine

Routines give the person with Alzheimer's disease some predictability and minimize confusion and disorientation. They provide a framework that is reassuring and helpful. Caregivers should also plan some time for themselves in their daily routine.

- Have meals at the same time every day.
- Plan activities such as walking, shopping, recreation, music, cooking, cleaning, day care, visitors, television and bedtime at regular times, as much as possible.
- Try to involve the person as much as possible in routine activities.
- Leave lots of time so the person is not rushed.

Adapt the Environment

It is important to create the right environment for people with Alzheimer's. They should be safe and have adequate space to move about and exercise. The area should be well lit, without too much glare or shadow. The temperature should be right; provide comfortable clothes that are not too hot or too cold. Create a walking circuit outside, so the person walks in a familiar area, on paths that always lead home again. A person with memory loss has problems understanding directions, and the fewer the choices, the fewer the chances of failure. Try to reduce clutter indoors, and leave rooms open, without moving furniture or familiar objects. Remove hazardous sharp objects, electrical appliances and dangerous tools.

Avoid surprises as much as possible. The slightest change can lead to confusion, frustration and irritability. Use lots of reminders—schedules, calendars, clocks and lists—to help the person remain oriented as much as possible. Simplify the environment by minimizing noise and people. Those with Alzheimer's do better one on one. They often cannot handle crowds, or conversations with more than two people at a time. Try to avoid problems in unfamiliar places by traveling with a few familiar people; keep out of crowds and noisy places.

Organize Activities

Don't involve the person in activities that will lead to over-stimulation, frustration or increased confusion. If a situation or environment is causing stress, remove the person gently. Calmly guide him or her away from the activity, in a reassuring voice. Use gentle touch to soothe the person—a back rub, a squeeze of the hand, a slow stroking of the hand or a shoulder massage.

Arrange exercise regularly: walking, swimming, cycling, dancing, tai chi, gardening, whatever the person prefers. Make it fun. Make sure activity is invigorating, not frustrating and tiring. Some people prefer small groups; others prefer to relate one on one and become confused and frustrated in groups.

Plan activities for when the person is rested. If it's a "bad" day, it may be wise to cancel activities that could cause problems, and take the day off. Try not to force the person to do something—wash, groom, wear certain clothes—if it is going to cause an argument. It may be better to leave the task undone for the day than to have a confrontation over it.

Communicate

Reasoning is the most commonly used mode of adult communication. In people with Alzheimer's disease, reasoning is impaired from the beginning. It is more useful to distract someone who is angry or agitated than to attempt to reason or deal head-on with the problem. Try a favorite food, music or a pleasurable activity. Gentle touching or massage, holding hands, hugging or quiet reading may be comforting and soothing for someone who is anxious, frustrated or angry. Remember that touching is one of the most basic human needs, and can be an effective method of communication.

Because of the language difficulties common in Alzheimer's, feelings, gestures and actions are even more important than words. Minimize distractions and communicate clearly at the person's level. Understand and learn to use nonverbal communication techniques. Make sure your nonverbal communication supports your verbal communication. Nonverbal cues include tone of voice, pitch and loudness, facial expression, touch, posture, eye contact and gestures. Allow lots of time for the person to listen and process the information you provide.

Ask questions that have yes or no answers, rather than open-ended or complicated questions. For example, don't ask, "What would you like for lunch?" or "Would you like a tuna sandwich or a tomato sandwich, a salad, soup and either milk,

---

Communicating with someone with Alzheimer's
- Make sure the person has his/her glasses and hearing aid.
- Reduce background noise and distractions.
- Use positive body language: relax, lean forward and smile.
- Touch the person gently and reassure him/her.
- Speak clearly and slowly.
- Give one idea at a time.
- Don't offer too many choices.
- Pause often and get feedback—"Is that okay?"
- Repeat your message as often as necessary.
- Distract the person if he/she becomes anxious or agitated.

coffee, tea or a soft drink?" Too many options are over-whelming; there is too much information to process. Instead try, "Would you like some lunch now?" (smiling and nodding). Give the person time to respond before you ask the next question. Maintain eye contact and smile before you proceed. "Would you like a sandwich?" (again smiling and nodding). Wait for a response. Then continue, "Would you like tuna in your sandwich?"

When you do give the person options, make sure they are easy to deal with. You want him or her to succeed. Present one idea at a time. Allow the person time to hear and process. Then allow time to respond. Better to get the communication right than to offer choices that will just lead to confusion.

Finding the right words to express thoughts can be a problem that frustrates both the person and the caregiver. Try "filling in the blanks" if you can, but change the subject or introduce diversion before frustration escalates.

In an Institution

For the most part, staff in institutions work hard and receive little appreciation. Many are extremely caring and dedicated. Communicate with the staff clearly. Ask them what you can do to help, and try to help as much as possible. Try to arrange to have the same staff with the person as often as possible. If the person does not get along with a particular staff member, for whatever reason, that staff member should not care for him or her, if at all possible. Work with the staff who get along best with the person.

Family should try to visit regularly to help out. If there is a problem at meals and the person likes company or needs help, visit at mealtime to lend a hand. If the person resists bathing, grooming or shaving, the family's presence at these times can be supportive. Family can even help with these tasks, or with giving medications if the person refuses to take them from the staff.

Prepare the person's biography for the staff so they know more and can use pet names or discuss topics of interest. A biography that includes photos and information about the person's experiences, hobbies and achievements can be made up on a large sheet of paper. This way someone with Alzheimer's remains a *person*, with family, interests and a career. The more information the staff have, the more successful they will be in communicating. Keep a log in the room to communicate with staff, family and friends. This will help to coordinate activities and keep everyone informed. Shift changes can be stressful and cause a lot of anxiety and confusion. Identify stressful times and develop strategies to smooth them over.

Managing Particular Behavior Problems

Memory

Understanding the Problem

Memory loss is the most common presenting feature in Alzheimer's disease. It is often the most frustrating, not only for the person but also for the caregiver. Try to understand the reason and nature of the memory loss (see chapter 3). Work with the memory that remains, and try to supplement what is lost. Because the person is unable to learn new information, understanding becomes much more difficult in any new environment or situation. There are many tricks you can use to help the person with poor short-term memory. Good caregivers attempt to find a balance between letting people try to the best of their ability and ensuring they do not fail. Do as little as possible and let the person do as much as possible.

Managing the Problem

- Establish rituals and routines around waking, meals, recreation, activities and bedtime to increase the sense of security and familiarity.
- Use memory aids, cues (verbal and written), calendars, lists, repetition of plans, reminders, backup information.
- Put the person's phone number and address in the wallet.
- Get a simple filing system.
- Set a routine and stick to it.
- Write down familiar phone numbers.
- Write out the plans for the day.
- Write out the weekly or daily menu.
- If people visit, keep the activity level low. Get them to come visit in a familiar place. Keep the noise level low and the numbers small.
- Constantly cue the person. Repeat information again and again until the person gets it. Give only bits of information at once. When the person becomes frustrated, shift to old memories.
- Reminisce by looking at family albums and videos. Old memories remain intact for a long time, and are a very positive way to connect with the person. Remember, he or she may feel isolated, frustrated and humiliated by memory losses. Any way you can connect in an affirming way is worthwhile.
- Teach family and close friends how to communicate. If they don't learn, they will avoid the person. They will find it too frustrating and depressing when they fail to connect with their loved one.
- Remind the person where money is stored for safekeeping. Take him or her there to point it out if he or she is looking for it.
- Help look for misplaced objects.

- Attach keys, purse or wallet to a belt so the person cannot misplace them.
- Do not scold the person for losing money, wallet or purse.
- Try to keep a spare set of keys or even an extra wallet in case one is lost.
- Learn where the person hides things.
- Investigate the person's concerns. Just because he or she has Alzheimer's does not mean that someone is not taking advantage. Make sure the person is not being abused by others.
- Use familiar activities as distractions: singsongs, painting, looking at photograph albums, playing cards, playing with pets, listening to music, having a massage or other simple activities. This allows the person to participate and have fun.
- Learn not to take accusations personally.

Repeating Questions and Stories

A family brought their aunt to the doctor for the first time. In the interview, the nephew said, "I thought we would never make it here." When he was asked why, he replied, "Because she phoned about forty times last night to ask about this appointment. She kept asking why she was coming, who arranged the appointment and what time we were picking her up."

Understanding the Problem

Repeating questions and stories is the hallmark behavior of Alzheimer's disease. If it is not present, it's not Alzheimer's. Often the first behavior to appear, it persists throughout the course of the illness. It stops only when the person loses the ability to express his or her thoughts. This behavior can be made a lot worse by stress, anxiety, depression and certain medications or illnesses.

A person who repeats a question again and again is stuck on one topic or idea and can't move on. Since the answer given is not *remembered*, the new information is not learned and the question is asked again. It's like having a song in your head that you can't get rid of.

Repeating a question is often the first sign of anxiety or agitation, and if it's allowed to persist the anxiety or agitation will escalate. A woman who can't express herself may keep asking urgently, "Where is the kitchen?" when in fact she is looking for the bathroom. Until her need to use the toilet is met, she will keep asking the same question, and will become more agitated about the caregiver's lack of understanding.

Ascertain what is driving the repeated question. Probe for the underlying problem. The woman at the doctor's was nervous because she didn't know why she was there. The family hadn't told her, or if they had, she'd forgotten. Different approaches could have put her mind at ease. The family could have asked what she was worried about; whether she was afraid she would have to stay in the hospital; whether she was afraid she would have to have an operation. Once she'd expressed her concerns, she could have been reassured. If she was unable to voice her fears, at least her overall anxiety could have been allayed.

Managing the Problem

Assess yourself as caregiver. How do the repeated questions make you feel? Are you angry, anxious, annoyed, frustrated (probably a little of all)? You need to center yourself, take control of your emotions and develop a plan.

Drop what you're doing until you gain control again. Try some deep breathing and clear your head. Develop your strategy in your mind and rehearse it for the next bout of questions. Practice what you will say. Bear in mind that the person asking the questions is worried and anxious and does not remember asking you the same question over and over. Focus on your own behavior and try different responses; make a game of discovering what works and what doesn't. Detach yourself; don't get caught up in the person's anxiety. Challenge yourself to remain in control. Become aware of your own voice; your tone and emotions will affect your responses. If you are still anxious, seek diversion or relaxation such as going out for a walk.

Other Do's

- Be patient and calm (this may require a conscious effort and learned techniques).
- Repeat the answer in simple words.
- Write down the answers to frequently asked or anticipated questions and leave them beside the person's phone if you don't live with him or her. Reading the information may satisfy the person and avoid another call to you.

Other Don't's

- Don't lose your cool or talk down to the person.
- Don't make the answer complicated.
- Don't tell the person too far in advance about visits to the doctor.
- Don't answer the phone if you are getting upset by all the calls. Get an answering machine and screen your calls until you are prepared to handle the situation.

Bathing and Dressing

People with Alzheimer's tend to develop problems with bathing and dressing at stage five (see the FAST chart earlier). Many resist help from caregivers because they want to bathe and dress themselves. These two problems are discussed together because the causes and coping strategies are similar.

Understanding the Problem

Problems with bathing and dressing may have physical or medical causes. Depression causes a person to lose interest in himself or herself. Physical illness, too, causes a loss of interest, energy and ability for self-care. Changes in the brain may also be responsible.

Environmental factors may be to blame. Lack of privacy, especially in an institution, may be an issue. Poor lighting will make it difficult for the person to see the tub or shower or items in the closet. The room may be too hot or cold, too noisy or uncomfortable.

Problems may occur for other reasons. The task may be too complicated or the person's attention span too short. The purpose of the task may have been forgotten. There may be a feeling of being forced by the caregiver. Fatigue may be a factor. The person may fear failing, or have general fear and anxiety.

Managing the Problem

Bathing: Choose the time of day when the person is the least agitated. This will avoid forcing him or her into the tub or shower. If the person becomes agitated, abandon your effort, wait for another time and try again. Be creative in the routines. Try cues such as turning on the spray as a warning that a shower is coming. Encourage the person to contribute to the routine as much as possible. Some people may be startled and afraid of the shower spray, and may prefer a leisurely, assisted tub bath. Ensure that the room is warm enough for comfort, and close the door and blinds to preserve privacy. Make sure that safety devices such as nonskid mats are secured. If these efforts to encourage the person are not enough, you can try giving a treat—whatever works. The bathroom should be prepared in advance, with everything organized and ready.

Bathing is a universal problem for people with Alzheimer's. If all efforts fail, offer baths more infrequently or choose bathing alternatives such as a sponge bath.

Dressing: Keep a routine for dressing, and avoid delays or interruptions in the process. Ensure that the room is warm enough for comfort, and close the door and blinds for privacy. If the person is able, allow some choice in clothes—for example, offer a blue blouse and a white blouse. Keep apparel simple—use pull-on tops and bottoms; avoid laces, zippers and buttons. Use Velcro and elastic. This may help to maintain the person's independence longer. Special clothing is available for Alzheimer's patients.

Anger, Aggression and Agitation

Mrs. Allen went to see the doctor in a wheelchair for an emergency visit. She had a black eye and bruises on her arm and chest, and was crying because, a few days before, her husband had lost control and had beaten her with his fists. She had no idea why he had done this. It came out of the blue. He just walked into the kitchen while she was making lunch and suddenly started shouting. When she told him to calm down, he began hitting her.

Mr. Allen is in the early stages of Alzheimer's. He has short-term memory loss and gets very frustrated when he cannot remember things. He is a neat person and likes to know where everything is.

Mrs. Allen described what happened in greater detail. She had just come home from the hospital about a week earlier, after a hip replacement for arthritis. While she was in the hospital, Mr. Allen stayed alone in the house and his daughter and homemakers made meals for him. Mrs. Allen left the hospital early because she didn't want him to be alone.

The day of the argument, she had asked him to go down to the basement to get chicken breasts from the freezer. He did and came back with beef. She sent him down again. This time he returned with bread. On the third attempt he came back up about fifteen minutes later with nothing. He kept forgetting what he was supposed to get, and when she reminded him he claimed there was no chicken in the freezer. He was becoming more and more agitated, and she was getting more and more frustrated. He started shouting at her, but she sent him down again anyway because she had to have chicken for lunch. Once more he insisted there was no chicken in the freezer. She sent him down for the fifth time. She was convinced he was too lazy to look for it, but because of her surgery she could not go downstairs herself to check. She thought he was doing it to annoy her and because he wanted beef for lunch, not chicken. This time he came up with beef again. When she told him she wouldn't cook the beef, he started shouting, she started shouting, and eventually he lost control and began hitting her.

She could not really understand what had happened. She was so upset about her hip, her pain and his anger. He did not remember the incident at all and had no idea how she got the bruises. She felt he was ungrateful, given that she had come home from the hospital early to take care of him.

Understanding the Problem

Mrs. Allen could have avoided this incident by trying to understand her husband's behavior in the context of his illness. She made a number of mistakes. First, she thought he was doing it to annoy her. She thought he was being deliberately stubborn. This is almost *never* the case. By asking him to do something he could not do, she set him up to fail again and again. When he failed, she chastised him. He got more and more frustrated each time he had to go up and down the stairs. Perhaps there really was no chicken in the freezer; perhaps her daughter had used it while Mrs. Allen was in the hospital. But it doesn't matter. She could have adapted to the situation and agreed to use the beef. She could have seen how her husband was becoming more and more agitated, and backed off. But she was in pain, frustrated and, as she said, "at the end of her tether." Her response made the situation worse and worse.

Aggressive behavior can range from irritability and agitation to verbal and even violent physical abuse. Caregivers are afraid and find this the most difficult behavior to manage. As many as 20 percent of people with Alzheimer's, and almost 50 percent of those living in institutions, show aggressive behaviors at times. Verbal aggression is almost twice as common as physical aggression. Aggression is more common among men, and is more common in certain forms of dementia. It is more common in frontal lobe dementia (see chapter 7) than in Alzheimer's disease.

There are stages of escalation before people become physically aggressive. Physical violence is usually the last stage. The table shows different phases of aggression, as well as suggestions for responses.

Aggression usually occurs when people are threatened, or think others are trying to harm them or steal from them, or when caregivers try to force them to do something. People are more likely to become aggressive when others try to provide intimate care—for example, bathing or toileting—or try to stop an intended activity—for example, wandering or going outside. People with Alzheimer's disease are also more likely to become irritable and angry, even aggressive, when they are tired or their routines are disrupted. If they wake at night and are disoriented or confused, they can become hostile and belligerent. Remember that they react in a wide variety of ways to pain, or even to discomfort from constipation or a full bladder.

Stages of aggression and suggested responses

Phases of aggression	Caregiver response
anxiety	active listening
restlessness and fidgeting	staying calm, friendly, amiable—trying to refocus attention
difficulty getting eye contact	unhurried concern
pacing, wandering, voice getting louder, speaking more quickly and interrupting	soothing and reassuring tone of voice
Stubborn and resistant	*Guiding and calming*
louder, resistant and challenging	clear, concise, simple responses
belligerent, threatening and challenging	setting limits, giving clear direction
clenched fists, inattentive	backing off
losing control	seeking help
aggressive action	self-protective action
loss of control	retreating
shouting, hitting, kicking, pushing, shaking, biting, lashing out	protecting self and others; restraining only if absolutely necessary, and with enough assistance
Aftermath	*Caring*
remorseful, exhausted, embarrassed, ashamed, withdrawn, sad, unaware of the aggressive event	recognizing behavior and triggers; release of tension is not necessarily directed at caregiver; forgiveness and support

Aggression can occur in a busy environment where there are too many strangers or noises, when people are surprised or startled, or if they are lost, insecure, forgotten, isolated, afraid of being abandoned or even jealous. They can take offense if the caregiver is insulting, irritable or abusive, or if the caregiver rushes them or makes them more frustrated by asking them to do tasks that they are no longer capable of doing.

People often become angry and irritable when they are overwhelmed because they have been given too much information. If they are given too many options at once or are asked too many questions that expose their problem and make them frustrated, anger results.

There is often a medical reason for people suddenly becoming aggressive. The first thing to do is to rule out a physical cause for the behavior. Certain medications, such as sedatives or antihistamines, may make people more angry and aggressive. This is called *disinhibition*—the person loses inhibitions and does things that he or she would otherwise not do. People who need aids such as glasses or hearing aids but don't use them are more likely to misinterpret the intentions of others because they do not correctly perceive, and therefore do not understand, what is happening around them. They may become frightened and feel threatened, and respond with aggression. If problems occur in the afternoon when the light starts to change—"sundowning"—turn on all the lights and sit the person under a light in a well-lit room. If they occur when he or she is asked to perform certain activities, get his or her hearing checked. Background noise from radio or television can result in problems with sound discrimination. Diminished hearing may result in speech being unintelligible, which can lead to misinterpretation and misunderstanding.

How the problem affects the person: Someone having an aggressive outburst may suffer an injury or hurt others. Rising blood pressure increases the risk of heart attack, stroke or injuries. The person says things he or she may not mean, and hurts the caregiver emotionally. After the outburst, the person feels exhausted.

How the problem affects the caregiver: Caregivers are often frightened and embarrassed when their loved ones become angry. They may feel a whole range of emotions from guilt (if they feel it was their fault) to anger, frustration, hurt, depression and hopelessness. Rage and physical aggression are the last straw for some caregivers. They may say, "Finally, that's it. Enough is enough. I'm not taking this anymore."

Managing the Problem

During an aggressive episode, approach the person gently and gain eye contact. Appear to be in control. Avoid gestures or postures that startle or can be interpreted as threatening, such as clenching your fists. Never turn your back on an overtly aggressive person. Retreat from the person's personal space and give lots of room. Avoid gestures such as pointing fingers or shouting. If you feel threatened, do not confront the person; just get out of the way. Never try to physically restrain an angry person. Walk beside or behind the person until the anger has subsided. Do not try to block him or her from going out a door; this will often make matters worse. If the person is threatening you, make sure there is no easy access to knives or other objects that could be used as weapons. Leave the scene if you feel at risk. Call neighbors, family, doctors or 911 for help.

When the episode is over, make notes on possible triggers for the aggression and the actions you took. Develop and test different strategies to prevent or reduce the behavior in the future. Later, the person may not even remember the episode and may think you are making it up. He or she may have a completely different perception from yours.

If the anger is frequent or violent, you will need to consult a doctor for treatment. Many different drugs are used to reduce or prevent violent behavior. If the person has delusions (you're not my wife, this is not my home, strangers are in the house, people are stealing things and so on) and is becoming aggressive or violent as a result, you will certainly need to seek treatment. People who have delusions are more likely to display aggressive behavior.

Other Do's

- Remember the person is most likely frustrated at the memory loss and confusion and is angry with the disease, not you.
- Try to settle the person with your voice, touch and expressions of love. Try soothing music, food, drinks, a hug or a kiss—anything you think might calm the person so the anger will pass more quickly.
- Avoid triggers you know will make the anger worse.

Other Don't's

- Don't get angry.
- Don't get caught up in the person's emotion.
- Don't try to argue or reason while the person is angry.
- Don't take responsibility for all problem behaviors.
- Don't feel guilty.
- Don't take the anger personally.

Delusions, Hallucinations and Paranoia

Mrs. Poulin brought Mr. Poulin to the clinic because she said he wanted to go "home" all the time. He got up at night and tried to kick her out of bed. He said his mother would come in and be angry if she found him in bed with a stranger.

Understanding the Problem

Delusions: People with Alzheimer's frequently think that their parents are still alive, that their spouses are not their spouses or that they are not living in their own houses. They demand to be taken home, often to a childhood home they have not visited for 50 years or more. Some believe their spouses are having affairs.

Managing sexual behaviors

Everybody needs to be touched, hugged and held, even people with Alzheimer's. Unfortunately, some of them are unable to express their needs in socially accepted ways. This leads to such behaviors as undressing in public, masturbating, touching others inappropriately, propositioning others or making sexual advances. To manage these problems, first, do not take offense. Remember, these people are often unaware of what they are doing. They may take their clothes off because they want to go to bed or to the bathroom, or because they are hot. Look for reasons for the behavior. Don't scold or ridicule the person but tell him or her gently that the behavior is not appropriate. Take the person to a private place or distract with food or activity. Be aware that some of your greetings or affectionate gestures may be misinterpreted and may encourage these behaviors.

Delusions, or mistaken belief in things that are not true, are not uncommon in Alzheimer's disease. They are firmly held, often in spite of obvious evidence to the contrary, and are usually resistant to persuasion or logic. The belief that someone is stealing money is a frequent delusion. For example, Mr. Poulin hid his money in the wardrobe. Then he claimed his son had stolen it. If he later found his money in the wardrobe, he might argue that his son had hidden it there, or returned it because he heard Mr. Poulin calling the police.

Hallucinations versus delusions: Hallucinations are sensory experiences that are not shared by others. In visual hallucinations people see things that are not there. In auditory hallucinations they hear things that are not there.

People with Alzheimer's often have visual and auditory hallucinations. More commonly, they misinterpret what they see or hear. For example, when watching a panel discussion on television they may begin to talk to the people on TV as if they were really in the room. When the show is over, they cannot understand where all the people have gone. Or they think they are much younger, or talk to photographs of dead husbands and other family members.

The most common hallucination is that there is a stranger in the house.

The Stranger in the Mirror

Recently a woman was taken to the doctor by her family because she kept complaining that there was a stranger in the house. Her family was advised to cover the mirrors, because when she looked in the mirror she did not recognize herself. She saw an old woman looking back at her, and the image was unfamiliar. Sure enough, when the family covered the mirrors the stranger disappeared.

A few months later the woman returned for a recheck and her daughter was asked about the stranger. She said it had happened only once since. The old lady had attended her granddaughter's wedding in a large city hotel and had gone to the ladies' room with her daughter to freshen up. When she went in, she looked into a huge mirror on the wall, pointing at the reflection. She gasped, "I knew you'd be here. I haven't seen you in a coon's age."

How the problem affects the person: Delusions and hallucinations add to the confusion of people with Alzheimer's disease. In some cases they are like a traveler stranded in a time warp. They have lost their memories of the last 20 years, and do not remember their children or moving to this new home or retiring. Now they live in this strange world, trying to make sense of it. No wonder they want to go home. They want to escape to a happier time when they were in control of their lives.

These delusions are common and they should be ignored, if at all possible. Reassure the person, but don't dwell on them. Only treat them with drugs if they are making the person angry, fearful or violent, or causing them to wander. If delusions are not associated with a behavior problem, just ignore them. For example, if a man with Alzheimer's occasionally says to his wife, Ann, when she comes into a room, "Where's Ann?" she can leave the room and return again. Chances are he'll recognize her and the next time say, "Ah, there you are." If the behavior continues, she can show him some recent photos of them together and gently reassure him that she is his wife. She can make a joke of it, blaming his eyesight or laughing it off, saying that she needs her hair done or looks so good because of a new dress.

How the problem affects the caregiver: Caregivers who do not know about delusions and hallucinations may actually believe the person, and think, for example, that people are coming in to steal things. Other caregivers may become alarmed and insist on treatment. It's important for caregivers to understand this behavior and the reasons behind it.

Paranoia: Paranoia results from impaired judgment that leads to unrealistic interpretations of the world. Others are blamed for actions that they did not commit. The person is convinced that people are trying to steal from or harm him or her, and cannot be dissuaded from this belief. No matter how hard caregivers attempt to explain or clarify the facts, people with Alzheimer's disease refuse or are unable to change their mind.

Managing the Problem

People who develop Alzheimer's become socially isolated because they have limited abilities to communicate and interact meaningfully with those around them. Family who are not recognized or are accused of stealing tend to avoid them, which further contributes to their isolation. They really need social support and the orientation other people provide. Avoidance just makes the matter worse.

As with aggressive behavior, first rule out a medical cause for the problem. Make sure that prescribed medications or over-the-counter drugs are not causing the problem or making it worse. Illness, infection, dehydration, pain, severe constipation or falls can lead to delusions and hallucinations, which are usually improved with appropriate treatment.

Remember that trying to reason or argue with the person may only reinforce the "unreal" world and the paranoia, increasing agitation, anger and confusion. For example, a man wakes up his caregiver at night and says he wants to go to visit his father. Instead of saying, "But your father has been dead for twenty years," try "You must miss him very much" or "You loved him very much." This opens up the conversation, allowing him to reminisce and express his feelings. If you reinforce reality by saying, "Your father is dead," he is cut off from his father. Let him discuss his feelings, even if he is confused about the facts. Validation of his feelings is more effective than reality orientation. You must meet him where he is, and not try to bring him into your reality. He cannot change. It's up to you to adapt.

Use music, exercise, pets, painting, drawing, reading, tapes, videos, photo albums, bird feeders, singalongs, visits to friends, cards and games to create a happy, relaxed mood and distractions. Ignore the delusions and hallucinations if at all possible. Don't take accusations personally. Remember, you can't get rid of them completely. The best you can aim for is a measure of control.

Other Do's

- Gloss over episodes of delusion, hallucination and paranoia. Chances are they will pass.
- Use humor if at all possible.
- Keep to routines.

- Turn the TV off or to a quiet nonviolent show; the voices may be confusing.
- Cover mirrors if there are "strangers in the house."
- Turn down the radio.
- Keep the environment free of clutter or distractions as much as possible.
- Keep a log of times and places where delusions and hallucinations occur. Try to find the triggers and remove them.

Other Don't's
- Don't try to convince the person he or she is wrong. Chances are that all your arguments will be forgotten; the same mistake will be made over and over again and this will just frustrate you.
- Don't get annoyed or angry.
- Don't think the person is doing it to annoy you.
- Don't scold.

Remember, too, that in some cases the person may be right. Check out his or her concerns, even if you suspect they are delusions. Many seniors are taken advantage of and abused. There are many people and organizations that prey on them, from the more legitimate businesses that confuse them by offering prizes if they send money, to out-and-out scams where they are asked for credit-card numbers and sold vacuum cleaners or services they do not need. Old or confused people are frequently victims of robbery or harassment. There may really be someone coming into the house and stealing things.

A Cautionary Tale
A man kept complaining to the manager of his apartment building about a huge snake living in his bathroom. He was

becoming more and more agitated. The Humane Society inspected the bathroom over and over, but found no sign of a snake. Eventually the man was institutionalized and given drugs and even electric shock treatment for his "delusions." While he was in the psychiatric institution, the manager of the building set about evicting him because the hospital staff felt it would be harmful to send him back to the same apartment. The manager was moving out his belongings when he walked into the bathroom and, lo and behold, there sat a six-foot boa constrictor. He screamed in fright. The boa slipped down the toilet and disappeared.

It turned out that the resident in the apartment below had the snake illegally in his bathroom. The boa regularly passed through the plumbing to the upstairs apartment, for a change of scenery.

Wandering

Wandering is common in Alzheimer's disease. Most people will wander at some time in some way. Random wandering occurs when a person moves about and does not know where he or she is going. In a secure area, this is not a problem. However, when people wander out in the street or in a hospital ward they may cause problems for themselves and others. Purposeful wandering occurs because people forget where they are or where they are going and want to escape. People wandering aimlessly in the community, often not dressed for the weather, are extremely vulnerable.

Understanding the Problem

People often wander because they cannot express their needs. For example, someone might want to go to the bathroom but not be able to express this wish. He or she might not even know what is wanted, and might become anxious, even agitated, walking about looking for whatever it is. Similarly, the wanderer may be driven by hunger, pain or constipation—or may just want to get out because a place feels strange and unfamiliar.

Environmental factors may contribute to the risk of wandering. The temperature may be too hot or too cold; the place may be too noisy or too quiet. Or the person may want to collect children from school, or go to work, based on distant memories that surface and become very real when recent memories are lost.

At night the person may wake up, not recognize the bedroom or house and leave to look for family or "home." He or she may be frightened by a dream or nightmare. Night wandering is very distressing for caregivers, who may sleep only lightly for years, for fear of their loved ones escaping. They may also, nightly, have to deal with an agitated person who is determined to escape.

Managing the Problem

The foremost consideration is the person's safety. Indoors and around the home, remove hazards and allow freedom to pace in the greatest possible space. To satisfy and control the urge to move about, take the person for walks around the neighborhood. Always travel in a circle so that the route inevitably leads home. Advise neighbors that the person has Alzheimer's so that if they ever see the person out alone, especially dressed inappropriately, they can call you or just fall in beside the person and gently lead him or her home.

Make sure the person gets adequate exercise. Remove items that may provoke the behavior: overcoats, outside shoes, umbrellas, walking sticks, purses, hats and so on. If these accessories are out of the way, the person may not think of going outside.

Anticipate physical triggers for wandering, such as hunger, thirst, the need to go to the bathroom, pain or anxiety. Learn to "read" restlessness, and experiment to find the right enticement to keep the person close to home—for example, food or a favorite physical activity. Note diversions that work, even only temporarily.

A comfortable environment is the most effective tool to coax the person to stay. Place familiar objects around the house to make it more homey and less threatening. Play familiar music. It may even be useful to put pictures on the doors of familiar rooms to prompt the person. For instance, put a picture of a toilet on the bathroom door, and of a bed on the bedroom door. The more confident and comfortable the person feels, the less likely you are to face problem behaviors.

Other Do's

- Enroll the person in the Wandering Person Registry in advance of any incident.
- Secure the home environment, including outdoor areas, to allow safe pacing, and provide for an alarm system if the person wanders away.
- Have the person carry identification whenever possible or, better yet, encourage wearing a medical alert bracelet inscribed "Memory Loss" or "Alzheimer's," with the Wandering Person Registry number.
- Activate the registry as soon as the person is missing, to start the police search promptly.
- Alert the neighborhood about a person at risk for wandering, and discuss possible approaches.
- Remain calm when the person is missing.
- Follow a pre-established step-by-step plan:

- quickly check the house/building, all exits, front and back property, and glance up and down the road and familiar routes the person may have taken;
  - call the Wandering Person Registry;
  - have on hand your relative's registration number and a current photograph;
  - recall what the wanderer is wearing;
  - follow police guidance;
  - call family members, neighbors and friends for help.
- Support and care for the wanderer when he or she returns.
- Try to keep the person awake and active during the day to ensure sleep at night. If you are up repeatedly at night, consult your doctor; a sleeping pill may help him or her get through the night.

Other Don't's

- Don't argue with the person or physically restrain him or her; it may lead to anger and aggression. If repeated redirection does not work, offer protective clothing and footwear, then walk along or follow at a distance.
- Don't secure the home with locks and bolts that you can't easily open in a hurry. Emergency personnel may need to get in quickly if something goes wrong.
- Don't panic when you can't find your relative. The majority of wanderers return on their own or are found in their neighborhood.
- Don't rush out on foot or by car to attempt a search yourself. The police can do a much better job; call them promptly. If the person returns and no one is at home, the wandering may resume.

SEVEN

Other Types of Dementia ·

Though there are over 60 recognized causes for dementia, by far the commonest is Alzheimer's disease, which accounts for about 60 percent of all cases. In another 15 to 20 percent, Alzheimer's occurs in people who have multiple small strokes as a contributing factor in their dementia. Thus 75 percent of the people who suffer from dementia have Alzheimer's, either alone or with these small strokes.

Atherosclerosis ("hardening of the arteries") of the brain's blood vessels, leading to multiple strokes, is the next commonest cause, and accounts for 15 to 20 percent of all cases. The remaining 5 to 10 percent result from a variety of degenerative diseases of the brain.

Stroke

Bill had been retired only a week when he suffered his first stroke. He'd felt quite normal the day before, and he and his wife had gone to bed at the usual time after playing bridge with friends. When Bill awoke the next morning, he couldn't get out of bed; he couldn't seem to get his right leg up and out from

Causes of dementia

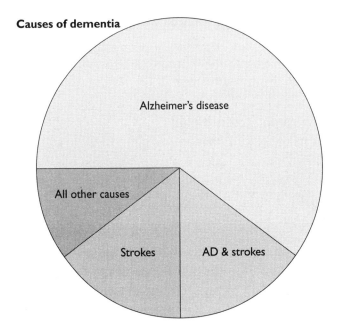

underneath the covers no matter how hard he tried. His right hand wouldn't work properly to lift the covers—it didn't hurt, but it didn't do what he wanted it to. He could see his hand flopping purposelessly at the end of his arm, useless and foreign. He tried to wake up his wife, who was lying beside him, but the name "Carol" didn't come out right. He could think of the name in his mind, but he couldn't get his mouth to make the sound, and all that came out was a garbled groan. He was eventually able to awaken her by shaking her with his good hand. She understood the situation right away and called an ambulance to take him to the hospital. The doctor confirmed that he had had a stroke and admitted him. Bill was in the hospital for the next three months, and after weeks of physiotherapy he was discharged home. He was able to walk only with a cane, and he had no use of his right hand. His speech was still garbled, but Carol could understand him.

Two months later Bill experienced what the doctor called a "ministroke." His face went numb one afternoon after lunch and his speech left him completely—he was only able to make unintelligible blowing sounds out of his flaccid mouth. He recovered, but he had two other similar "ministrokes" over the next two weeks. Carol felt that he was never quite the same afterward. She noted that he was more irritable and less thoughtful. He seemed to get frustrated easily and burst into tears at the slightest difficulty. She could feel him withdrawing emotionally from her, and though she tried to be cheerful, sometimes in the evening he would sit in his wheelchair, looking out the window, silently crying.

She said she felt it was as if he were dying bit by bit, from the top down.

What a Stroke Does

A stroke is a sudden loss of brain function caused by an interruption of the blood supply to some area of the brain. Usually painless, a stroke comes on swiftly (hence the name) and often without warning. The affected part of the brain no longer works properly—it doesn't do what it used to do only a few minutes before. The symptoms and signs of the stroke depend on which area of the brain is involved. Strokes can be massive and rapidly fatal, but they can also produce very subtle changes. Bill's stroke produced weakness in his right hand and leg, as well as difficulty in speech—a common pattern—but strokes may also produce weakness of the eyes or face, difficulties in memory or insight, dizziness and unsteady gait, confusion, inappropriate behaviors, or any other neurological problem, including dementia.

A stroke happens when the normal blood flow to an area of the brain is cut off, causing the cells in that part of the brain to die. Strokes most commonly occur when arteries that have already been narrowed by atherosclerosis (the buildup of fatty substances in the lining of the artery) become completely blocked. Either the lining of the artery becomes so built up that no blood can get through, or *emboli*, tiny pieces of material, catch on the irregular surface of the narrowed vessel and block it off.

Though most strokes are caused by blockage of an artery, some result when atherosclerosis weakens the wall of the blood vessel to the point where the blood vessel bursts and blood hemorrhages into the tissue of the brain. In this instance the escaped blood in the brain tissue damages the cells and causes them to die.

Whether the brain cells die from a lack of blood supply, or from hemorrhage, the result is much the same; the part of the brain affected no longer functions properly. The proper medical term to describe a stroke is "cerebrovascular accident" (brain-vessel accident).

Multi-Infarct (Vascular) Dementia

When blood flow is interrupted and cells die, the process is called *infarction*. If the area involved is a part of the brain responsible for memory or insight, these functions will no longer be normal. If several small arteries in the brain are damaged, there are multiple infarcts. Alzheimer's disease cannot be diagnosed unless *multi-infarct dementia* (also called *vascular* [blood-vessel] *dementia*) is ruled out. Clinically, this dementia differs from Alzheimer's in several ways. Rather than having a gradual onset, it often starts with a specific event (the initial stroke) and progresses in steps over months or years as further strokes occur. Sometimes, because the strokes have been relatively tiny, the person has not noticed any sudden loss of a particular brain function, but only the general mental decline of dementia, indistinguishable from Alzheimer's disease. Both conditions can produce poor intellectual functioning, poor reasoning and calculating ability and poor memory. (In anatomical terms, you need to damage between 50 and 100 mL of brain tissue to produce dementia, but often damage to as little as 10 mL can worsen intellectual functioning.) On a CT scan of multi-infarct dementia, the small areas where brain cells have died can be seen as vacant spaces or holes called *lacunae* (from the Latin for "lake").

Binswanger's disease is a form of dementia caused by chronic reduced blood flow in the brain's white matter, leading to scarring of the white matter. It may be associated with multiple small infarcts and is often seen in people with high blood pressure.

The Dementia of Down Syndrome

Down syndrome is a genetic disorder first described in 1886, by the English physician Dr. John Langdon Down. People with this syndrome inherit an extra chromosome and this causes limitations in their physical and intellectual development. The syndrome occurs once in every 700 births. The cause of the

Causes of multi-infarct dementia

Since most strokes result from atherosclerosis weakening the artery wall and predisposing the artery to blockage or hemorrhage, any risk factor for atherosclerosis—such as high blood cholesterol, smoking, high blood pressure, diabetes—increases the risk of stroke. Brain hemorrhage is more common in those who have high blood pressure, and emboli are commonly seen in those with irregular heartbeats, especially atrial fibrillation. It is important to recognize this cause of dementia because attention to the risk factors for atherosclerosis can stop the dementia from progressing—as opposed to Alzheimer's disease, where we are powerless to prevent worsening of the condition. In addition, 20 percent of people with Alzheimer's also have multiple small strokes that could contribute to their poor intellectual functioning.

Poor blood flow to the brain

In Alzheimer's time, physicians believed that most of the feeblemindedness of old age was caused by poor blood flow to the brain—a sort of strangulation of this essential organ. We now know that this is not the case. Most people with pure Alzheimer's disease have no significant problem with cerebral blood flow. However, poor blood flow to the brain can cause brain damage (such as strokes) and even dementia. Usually, strokes produce significant local signs (such as the weakness in Bill's case). However, these signs very much depend on the amount of brain tissue damaged and the site. It is possible to have "silent" strokes—that is, repeated damage to small areas of the brain whose loss of function is not readily appreciated. These multiple small strokes are often cumulative in their damage, and though each individual one is not noticed, the total effect is that the brain does not work well, resulting in dementia. The person may complain of memory loss, show poor insight or planning skills, or may be unable to do what he or she could do before—many of the symptoms of Alzheimer's—but the underlying cause is the cumulative damage to brain cells from interruptions to their blood supply.

---

extra chromosome is not known, but the risk of inheriting the disease increases directly with the age of the mother at the time of birth.

Almost all people with Down syndrome who live past the age of 35 develop changes in their brains identical to those of Alzheimer's disease, including the plaques and neurofibrillary tangles. In one study, the brains of 90 percent of people with Down syndrome who had died at age 30 or older showed these changes. Yet not all these people had become demented—that is, not all had the loss of memory and the reasoning abnormalities usually seen in Alzheimer's disease. This may have been because 65 percent of those with Down syndrome have a markedly reduced IQ—in the range of 20 to 50, compared with a normal IQ of around 100—and standard psychological testing may not be as effective at picking up mental deterioration in them as in people of average intelligence. Many people with Down syndrome do deteriorate mentally as they age: they may lose the ability to care for themselves; their language and communication skills may decline; they may withdraw and become less interested in social interaction; they may wander; and they may become difficult or even unmanageable in their behavior—all typical findings in Alzheimer's disease. However, only 30 to 50 percent of those over age 35 show this kind of mental deterioration, in spite of the fact that 90 percent show typical Alzheimer's changes in their brains. For some unknown reason, there are people with Down syndrome who have little change in their mental abilities despite these neuropathological signs.

The evidence clearly points to a link between Down syndrome and Alzheimer's disease. What the link is, and why people with Down syndrome sometimes seem to escape further mental impairment, remains unclear.

The Dementia of AIDS

Infection with the AIDS virus (HIV) can produce a dementia referred to as "AIDS dementia complex." Most people with AIDS dementia complex have overt AIDS—that is, they have the signs and symptoms of decreased immunity—by the time the mental changes become evident. However, in almost 20 percent the mental changes are the first signs that something may be wrong.

There is markedly decreased resistance to infection of all types in AIDS, and infections with opportunistic organisms such as fungi, bacteria and other viruses can produce distinct alterations in brain function. Thus, the diagnosis of dementia in AIDS is not straightforward. In typical cases of AIDS dementia complex, however, people develop forgetfulness and poor concentration as well as slowed thought processes and speech.

They become apathetic and withdrawn and their mental difficulties usually progress slowly, with indifference and quiet confusion being the typical course. A small number of people develop agitation and psychosis.

The dementia of the AIDS complex is often improved by the use of specific antiviral drugs directed against the AIDS virus.

Hydrocephalus

The brain and spinal cord are both suspended in a thin liquid called *cerebrospinal fluid*, which nourishes and protects these vital organs. This fluid is produced within the brain, and percolates through a complicated system of tubes and chambers to bathe the tissues and then be reabsorbed. Any obstruction in the flow of this liquid can cause excessive accumulation in the brain, a condition called *hydrocephalus* (from the Greek meaning "water" and "head").

In a newborn infant this increased amount of liquid within the brain can distend the still pliant skull bones, and the head may be quite large. In adults, however, excess cerebrospinal fluid usually accumulates gradually, without changes in the external appearance of the skull. The increased pressure can produce a dementia with behavior indistinguishable from that of Alzheimer's by interfering with normal brain function.

Adult hydrocephalus produces three common symptoms:

- Unsteadiness of gait and balance, with the greatest difficulty on stairs and curbs; frequent falls; wide-based walking and weakness in the legs. This may be progressive and may eventually prevent walking altogether.
- Incontinence of urine, which often begins with a sense of bladder urgency—a sudden feeling of having to urinate—followed by loss of control of urination. Later, total incontinence and even indifference to the incontinence may develop.

• Dementia, indistinguishable from the behavior in Alzheimer's disease, resulting from the excess pressure on the brain.

A CT scan usually allows diagnosis of hydrocephalus, as the abnormal collections of fluid can be seen quite easily. Not all hydrocephalus is reversible, but many people have their dementia improve or even disappear completely when the excess fluid is drained and the pressure is reduced.

Pick's Disease

In the early part of this century, a Czech psychiatrist named Arnold Pick described several cases that he had seen in his practice in Prague. All his patients had a rapidly progressive dementia, but their disease differed from the illness discovered by his colleague Dr. Alzheimer in that they seemed to be much more emotionally unstable, with early changes in their personality, and they seemed to show much more disinhibition early in the course of the disease. They were often brought to the psychiatrist because of some event showing very poor judgment or some behavior simply not acceptable to society. Dr. Pick noted that the speech of many of these people was just a medley of disconnected words and phrases. Their moods were extreme. Some seemed to be apathetic and withdrawn; others were the exact opposite—unduly jocular and manic. Dr. Pick felt that this group of people might represent a different type of dementia from that described by Dr. Alzheimer.

When the brain tissues of these people were examined at autopsy, they did prove to differ significantly from the brain tissues of those with Alzheimer's disease. Marked atrophy (shrinkage) of the brain was present, but this shrinkage was not evident throughout the entire brain, as in advanced Alzheimer's disease; rather, it was limited to only two areas of the cortex: the frontal lobe and the temporal lobe. The brain in Pick's disease is often very thin in these areas—much thinner than that seen in Alzheimer's; indeed, it has been described as "paper-thin—like the kernel of a dried walnut." Curiously, the thinning stops abruptly, leaving relatively unspared brain right next door. In addition, Dr. Pick noted that the changes in this disease occurred throughout the whole thickness of the frontal and temporal lobes—unlike Alzheimer's, which affects only the outer layer, the cortex. Under the microscope, neurofilaments can be seen within the cells of the brain, just as in the brain tissue of people with Alzheimer's. However, in Alzheimer's disease the neurofilaments are twisted in a helical fashion, whereas in Pick's disease the filaments are straight. Senile plaques can also be seen in Pick's disease, but not nearly in the number seen in Alzheimer's.

We now realize that Pick's disease is a completely separate malady from Alzheimer's disease. It accounts for only 1 to 2 percent of all dementias, is more common in women and seems to progress more rapidly in younger people. The cause is not known. There is some evidence of a genetic tendency.

Often it is impossible to differentiate Pick's disease from Alzheimer's disease except at autopsy, as the symptoms and signs are too similar. Because the frontal lobe is more involved in Pick's disease, signs and symptoms of frontal lobe abnormality are more commonly seen. The frontal lobe is responsible for insight, social graces and tact, and it controls or filters the emotions. Accordingly, many people with Pick's disease have deteriorating social skills early in the course of their disease. They are less tactful, make poor social judgments, are less inhibited and have changes in their personality. They have problems with sexuality—such as inappropriate sexual activity, exhibitionism, unrestrained use of sexual phrases or even promiscuity. Mood changes are often marked—from apathy to wild euphoria. The deterioration in character and social functions appears before the other changes of dementia, including memory loss. These people show poor planning skills and goal achievement. Language changes are prominent early on, and language quickly deteriorates.

The distinct shrinkage of the frontal and temporal lobes can be seen on a CT scan or MRI, but a certain diagnosis is usually made only at autopsy.

Frontal Lobe Dementia

Only over the past several years has this dementia been described and diagnosed as a new disease. It seems to be a variant of Alzheimer's, with marked shrinkage of the frontal lobe but without the cellular changes seen in Pick's disease. Thus, it appears to be a mix of the two diseases, with features of both. It is much more common than Pick's disease.

People with frontal lobe dementia are often younger when their symptoms begin, and because atrophy of the frontal lobe is the characteristic brain damage, they usually show progressive change in their personalities and breakdown in their social conduct. They often have poor personal hygiene, markedly reduced initiative and insight and a general loss of concern or sympathy for others (especially their families). Their behavior often becomes rigid and inflexible, with repetition of simple tasks such as hand washing, rhythmic clapping, or emptying and then refilling a handbag. They cannot understand why they perform these acts repetitively, but they become quite emotionally upset if interrupted. They seem unaffected by the concern of others. Often they change their eating patterns: they may overeat, or limit their diet to a small number of foods.

In contrast to Alzheimer's disease, memory is relatively well preserved, and these people have very little visual or spatial disorientation. Language abnormalities are not prominent early on, though a gradual loss of language function usually

The edible dementia

In 1957, Dr. Carlton Gajdusek stunned the scientific and medical world with his study of a mysterious progressive brain disorder that was transmitted by cannibalism.

The disease was found in the eastern highlands of the island of New Guinea, among the members of a Stone Age tribe called the Fore. The rapidly fatal dementia was common among women and children in the mountainous region, and the Fore people believed that it was the result of magic worked upon the victim by an enemy. It began with difficulty walking—an unsteadiness of gait—and then quickly progressed to a shaking or trembling of muscles, with slurring of speech and increasing weakness. The Fore called it *kuru*—a word that in their language means the shivering or trembling associated with fear or cold. The disease relentlessly progressed to loss of muscle coordination and power, leaving its victims unable to stand or even sit unattended. Speech became unintelligible; incontinence of both bowel and bladder followed; and then, mercifully, came coma and death—usually within 6 to 12 months of the onset of the trembling. Gajdusek proved that kuru was caused by an infection; tissue from a victim's brain was injected into a chimpanzee, and 18 months later the laboratory animal developed the disease.

In the Fore culture, elders were highly respected, and it was the custom to eat the bodies and brains of the deceased to gain their knowledge and experience. Women and young children were responsible for preparing the dead body, a task that included opening the skull, removing the brain and cooking it ritualistically. This allowed ample opportunity for the infectious organisms to be absorbed by the mourners—either by being eaten or through contact with skin openings such as sores or mucous membranes during preparation of the dead tissue. Thus, the dreaded disease was passed from generation to generation by the funerary rites of cannibalism.

There have been no new cases of kuru since the practice of ritualistic cannibalism was stopped. The infectious organism has never been isolated, but kuru has been transmitted in experiments to all sorts of animal hosts, including sheep, goats, calves, mink, cats, raccoons, mice and rabbits. The usual method of transmission in these experiments is to take a small amount of infected brain and inject it directly into the brain of the experimental animal. However, experiments have also been done to prove that kuru can be transmitted by contaminated food. In one experiment, small pieces of kuru-infected chimpanzee brain were mixed into the food of a healthy chimpanzee. Months later, the chimpanzee developed kuru, proving that the disease could be transmitted by food—an edible dementia.

occurs as the disease progresses. Unlike people with Alzheimer's, these people's social skills and insights seem to be much more severely affected than their mental function in general, so their ability to calculate and reason is relatively well preserved until late in the disease.

About 50 percent of people with frontal lobe dementia have a close relative with dementia.

Parkinson's Disease

The English physician James Parkinson first described this common disorder in 1817. Parkinson's disease produces a characteristic tremor at rest, rigid movement and decreased mobility, with a shuffling gait. It is a progressive deterioration of specific areas in the base of the brain, resulting in loss of the neurotransmitter *dopamine*. It affects about 1 percent of the population over age 50, and up to 30 percent of people with Parkinson's disease will eventually develop dementia. Those who develop the dementia are often disoriented at night, with visual and auditory hallucinations.

The signs and symptoms of Parkinson's disease are to some extent treatable with dopamine, the neurotransmitter that is reduced by the disease process. Accordingly, dementia in someone with Parkinson's may be improved by use of the drug. Also, because depression is common in Parkinson's disease, antidepressants are often helpful.

Dementia with Lewy Bodies (DLB)

Lewy body dementia is named after the pathologist Fredrich Lewy, who first described Lewy bodies—flecks of dense material—in the cells of the brains of people who had dementia. There is a great deal of overlap between the different dementias. About a quarter of the people who have been diagnosed with Alzheimer's disease have Lewy bodies in their brains,

"Punch-drunk"—dementia pugilistica

Forgetfulness, slowness in thinking and deterioration in speech are often seen in boxers as they age. These are caused by repeated blows to the head. Though each single blow may not produce a large area of damage within the brain, over the years the accumulated scars destroy enough brain tissue to impair mental function and produce the symptoms of dementia. Similarly, repeated head injuries from any other cause (for example, car accidents) can produce alterations of brain function and even dementia. The problem is similar to that of multi-infarct dementia, in which multiple small strokes are cumulative in effect. In boxers, Parkinsonian symptoms of tremor and rigidity are often present and the gait may be unsteady. In one study, fully half the professional boxers tested showed abnormalities on a CT scan, and the number of brain scars was directly related to the number of professional bouts the boxer had fought. The scar tissue is distributed diffusely throughout the brain. Dementia pugilistica (fighters' dementia) shows neurofibrillary changes typical of Alzheimer's, but senile plaques (such an important part of the diagnosis of Alzheimer's) are not present.

In several large studies, head injuries—whether suffered during boxing matches or not—have been associated with an increased risk of Alzheimer's disease, but the data are not consistent. It is possible that repeated blows to the head, causing microscopic damage, may initiate some or all of the changes of Alzheimer's, or at least predispose the person to such changes in some way. However, though dementia pugilistica may have some similar features, it is definitely not identical to Alzheimer's disease.

and about half the people who have Parkinson's disease have changes in their brains that are consistent with Alzheimer's disease. Many people who have Parkinson's disease also have Lewy bodies in their brains.

People who have dementia with Lewy bodies have some fairly characteristic features. Many have features of Parkinson's. Their movement is slower than normal. Their muscle tone is increased, so they are stiff. In fact, slow movements and rigidity are the most common signs. They also tend to fall and to have *fluctuating cognition.*

Normally, people with dementia get more confused in late afternoon and evening (sundowning). People with DLB have individual episodes of confusion that can last for minutes or hours. They have good days and bad days. They also fluctuate in alertness and attention. At times they "go blank." Some are drowsy, sleepy, withdrawn and mumbling. They have episodes where they are "out of it," stare blankly or "lose it," making no sense. They can have visual hallucinations in which they see animals, children and insects. They often have well formed and detailed delusions (e.g., spouse having an affair, people in the house). If the rigidity and slowness come first, the condition is called Parkinson's disease. If the memory loss comes before the physical symptoms, the condition is called DLB.

These people often do not respond well to anti-Parkinson's medications. They become depressed more often than people with Alzheimer's. They often respond well to cholinergic drugs like rivastigmine, galantamine and donepezil.

Features of DLB

Major
- fluctuating cognition, with changes in attention and alertness
- recurrent visual hallucinations, well formed and detailed
- slowed movement, stiffness, (can't get out of chair or turn in bed, shuffle while walking, etc.)

Minor
- falling
- passing out
- transient loss of consciousness, "out of it," "going blank and staring into space"
- sensitive to neuroleptics (e.g., haloperidol, see chapter 10)
- delusions (spouse having an affair, people trying to harm them, etc.)

- hallucinations of touch (e.g., somebody in bed), or smell (e.g., water has peculiar smell)

Someone with two of the major features above has probable dementia with Lewy bodies. Someone with one of these major features has possible DLB.

Probable and Possible Dementia with Lewy Bodies
People with probable and possible DLB have progressive cognitive decline that impairs their ability to function independently. They have poor attention and impaired visuo-spatial ability.

Creutzfeldt-Jakob Disease

In the spring of 1913, a 23-year-old German maid named Bertha was taken to the University Hospital in the town of Breslau, Germany, where Dr. Alois Alzheimer was chief neurologist. She had experienced a dramatic change in her personality over the previous few weeks and was behaving strangely. She didn't see the renowned Dr. Alzheimer but was examined by one of his young assistants, Dr. Hans Gerhard Creutzfeldt, who reported that she "no longer wanted to eat or bathe, neglected her appearance and became dirty. She assumed particular postures." The visit had been prompted by the fact that, several days earlier, she had "suddenly screamed out that her sister was dead and that she was to blame ... and that she wanted to sacrifice herself." Dr. Creutzfeldt examined Bertha and found evidence of spasticity in her legs, a shaking tremor that incapacitated her whenever she tried to move and a curious oscillation of mood between agitation and apathy. In spite of her obvious problems, she had frequent "unmotivated outbursts of laughter." The woman was admitted to the hospital and rapidly developed all the signs of dementia as well as epilepsy. She died during an epileptic seizure. The whole disease process had lasted less than six months.

At autopsy, Dr. Creutzfeldt found a "marked fall out of the gray cells everywhere within the brain," and strange, vacant-looking empty holes, or *vacuoles*, where the neurons had once been. The resulting empty spaces in the brain made the organ resemble a huge sponge.

The year after Dr. Creutzfeldt described Bertha's case in the medical literature, a colleague of his at the University of Hamburg, Dr. Alfons Jakob, described several more cases of this rapidly progressive dementia that caused so much neuron loss. The new disease was given the scientific name "subacute spongiform encephalopathy."

Creutzfeldt-Jakob disease, as it has come to be known, is an uncommon cause of dementia, and only about 3,500 cases have ever been diagnosed. In Canada, 334 deaths were attributed to Creutzfeldt-Jakob disease in the 15 years from 1979 to 1993—about 20 a year. The prevalence of the disease is between .45 and 1 per million population worldwide, and it affects all races in all climates. It accounts for about 200 cases of dementia in the United States each year. Some 10 to 15 percent of the cases have a family history of the disorder.

The dementia may begin suddenly, but often the first complaints are a vague dizziness and weakness, rapidly followed by difficulties in coordination, walking and vision. Memory loss is always present, and poor judgment follows soon thereafter. Rigidity and tremors restrict mobility early. Blindness is seen in about half the cases and emotional instability is usual. Muscle jerking is characteristic, particularly when the person is startled—this produces a sudden, uncoordinated jerking of many muscle groups. Even at rest, the fine twitching of various muscle fibers can often easily be seen. The person looks to be very cold and shivering. The dementia rapidly progresses to

Mad cow disease

In 1985, veterinarians in the United Kingdom recognized several cases of a new and unusual type of brain degeneration in dairy herds. The affected cows all had decreased milk production, were unsteady in standing or walking and became irritable and unpredictable in their behavior. Cows are usually docile creatures, so dairy farmers called these cows "mad" because of their aggressive temperament. The new disease was attributed to the use of sheep brains as food for the cows, a practice initiated in the late 1970s in Britain. Cows usually get their protein from grasses and grains, and the sheep's brains had been added to the feed as an extra source of protein, much as ground-up fish meal is sometimes used; it seemed like a good idea to use the protein instead of simply disposing of it.

Unfortunately, sheep have long been known to have their own particular type of dementia, called "scrapie." The name comes from the behavior of infected sheep, which become irritated and itchy and rub up against fence posts, trees or brush so vigorously that they often scrape their wool completely off. Infected sheep also have difficulty walking, and stagger, will not eat and eventually go blind and die. Scrapie can be easily transmitted to other animal species, though the infectious agent has never been identified. Veterinarians feared that feeding sheep brains infected with scrapie to cows might have transmitted scrapie to the cows. In addition, the temperature at some of the rendering plants (rendering is the process of melting down all the usually unused parts of animal carcasses) had been reduced, and the process of extracting the fat had been altered. It was possible that the lower temperature and the new chemical techniques of removing fat had allowed the infectious agent for scrapie to survive the rendering plant and produce the disease.

Soon the number of cases of mad cow disease in the United Kingdom rose dramatically—up to 37,000 a year, compared with 150 cases a year in the rest of Europe—and in 1988 the government banned the use of ruminant tissue (including sheep's brains) as feed. Mad cow disease is an infectious dementia, and it has been shown that it can be transmitted from cows to various other animal species including pigs.

Unfortunately, several dairy workers, all of whom had been exposed to mad cow disease, developed what seemed to be Creutzfeldt-Jakob dementia, and because mad cow disease had been transmitted to other animal species, there was concern that the disease had spread from cows to their handlers.

Events took an ominous turn in March 1996, when ten cases of a new variant of Creutzfeldt-Jakob disease were diagnosed in Britain. This new variant affected much younger people, began with psychiatric symptoms but rapidly progressed to dementia and death and, most significantly, caused changes in the brain that characterized it as medically different from classic Creutzfeldt-Jakob disease, though related to it. The suspicion is that this new disease is mad cow disease that has jumped the species barrier from cows to humans. But no direct proof of this exists, and no one knows for sure whether contact with infected cows or eating their meat can cause dementia in humans.

Only one case of mad cow disease has been recorded in Canada, and that was in an animal imported from the United Kingdom. There has never been a single "mad cow" in the U.S.A.

Should you eat beef? In Canada and the U.S., there is no evidence that eating beef poses a threat for the development of dementia. In the United Kingdom, the question can't be answered with certainty, but many suggest that there is a risk (albeit a very small one) of acquiring dementia from infected animal parts.

complete disability and a vegetative state, with death often occurring within a year.

Creutzfeldt-Jakob dementia is infectious. Brain tissue taken from people with the disease and injected into chimpanzees can produce the dementia after an incubation period of a year or longer. The disease has also been transmitted to other primates, as well as cats, pigs, mice and even guinea pigs. Yet not all species inoculated have contracted the disease. The infectious agent has not been identified, but there are records of Creutzfeldt-Jakob disease being transmitted from human to human by corneal transplantation, by neurosurgical instruments shared by patients and by the injection of human growth hormone collected from brains infected with the disease. There has never been documentation of a case transmitted by blood transfusion. The disease is not easily transmitted, and spouses and other close contacts do not have an increased incidence of the dementia. No evidence exists that stool, urine, saliva or other secretions can transmit the disease.

Recently, a new variant of Creutzfeldt-Jakob disease has been identified in several people in the United Kingdom and France. Though Creutzfeldt's original case, Bertha, was only 23, the disease usually affects people in their fifties or sixties. This new variant affects much younger people (the average age was only 27) and has several pathological differences from the classic disease described years ago. These new variants may be related to the incidence of bovine spongiform encephalopathy (BSE), the condition popularly known as "mad cow disease."

EIGHT

What Causes Alzheimer's Disease?

eredity doubtlessly plays a very important role in Alzheimer's. Although not all the details are understood thus far, heredity appears to be the only cause for Alzheimer's that occurs at an early age. However, in the vast majority of Alzheimer's cases—those appearing after the age of 60—two groups of factors seem necessary to produce the disease: a genetic predisposition, and some other factor or factors such as inflammation, exposure to toxins such as aluminum, viral infections and so on. Certainly we have a lot to learn about how Alzheimer's develops.

Heredity

In some families, it has been observed that half the members develop typical Alzheimer's disease at a relatively young age (in their forties or fifties) and the disease may be traced over several generations. This so-called familial Alzheimer's disease accounts for only 5 to 10 percent of the total number of cases, but this particular type of Alzheimer's has been shown to be

Can wine prevent Alzheimer's?

A study in Bordeaux, France, suggested that drinking wine may be associated with a decreased incidence of Alzheimer's disease. In this study of 3,700 people over age 65, the greatest incidence of Alzheimer's appeared in those who did not drink at all or drank less than one glass of wine a week. In contrast, those who drank between two and four glasses of wine a day were found to have a significantly reduced incidence. In a recent study in Rotterdam, researchers found that people who drank three drinks every day were 40 percent less likely to develop Alzheimer's than people who did not drink. However, researchers emphasize that a cause-and-effect relationship has not yet been established, and warn that excessive alcohol use carries its own risk of medical problems. Current research suggests that alcohol use should not exceed three drinks per day. One drink is defined as 5 ounces (142 mL) of wine, 12 ounces (341 mL) of beer, 1.5 ounces (45 mL) of liquor or 3 ounces (90 mL) of fortified wine such as port or sherry. Safe drinking limits are affected by certain medications and physical conditions. If in doubt, consult your doctor.

entirely inherited. The gene defect can be passed on to either male or female in the next generation, and will cause the brain degeneration typical of Alzheimer's in the 50 percent of the children who inherit it. Recently, researchers discovered that an abnormality on chromosome 14 is present in 70 percent of the families with this type of familial Alzheimer's. Gene defects on chromosome 21 and chromosome 1 are also associated with this form of the disease. Thus, this form of Alzheimer's appears to stem from a genetic defect that by itself produces the disease.

For the more common type of Alzheimer's—where there is no clear-cut high incidence of disease in the family and where the symptoms come on later in life—the role of genetics is felt to be contributory but not as dominant. Having a brother or sister, parent or child with late-onset disease (after age 65) increases your risk by 3.5 to 4 times, but there seem to be other

Does smoking protect against Alzheimer's?

Many large studies have shown that cigarette smokers are approximately 50 percent less likely to develop Alzheimer's disease than nonsmokers. This may not be a cause-and-effect relationship—that is, the smoking itself may not decrease the risk of Alzheimer's but may simply be associated with some other factor that decreases the risk.

Nicotine, one of the most powerful chemicals in cigarette smoke, has been shown to improve cognitive performance in normal healthy adults and in people with Alzheimer's disease. How it does so is not clear, but it may facilitate neurotransmitter action. Nicotine may have a direct effect as a neurotransmitter itself, improving the communication between nerve cells, or the presence of nicotine may increase the release of other neurotransmitters such as acetylcholine. In addition, the receptors for nicotine increase in the brain with chronic use of the drug (such as smoking). We know that nicotine receptors in the brain are decreased in Alzheimer's disease, so perhaps smokers, because they have increased their nicotine receptors through their years of smoking, are less affected by the ongoing loss. (Cigarette smoking has also been associated with a decreased risk of Parkinson's disease.)

Unfortunately, cigarette smoking has disastrous health consequences (chronic lung disease, heart disease, stroke, various cancers, etc.) It cannot be recommended as a way to decrease the risk of Alzheimer's.

factors that are important, as well. Identical twins share exactly the same genetics, yet if one of the twins develops late-onset Alzheimer's, there is an 80 percent chance that the other twin will also. Thus, some factor other than genetics must be playing a role. Separating the role of genes from the role of nongenetic factors such as toxic agents, viruses, inflammation, head injury and so on is very difficult, and the relationship is not completely understood. It may be that heredity only makes someone susceptible, and that a particular trigger is necessary before the disease develops.

Specific Chromosomal Abnormalities

- *Chromosome 21*: This chromosome was suspected of being

Beta amyloid protein

In an attempt to understand the causes of Alzheimer's disease, brain researchers have focused on the telltale signs of the disease: the neuritic (senile) plaques and the neurofibrillary tangles. They have discovered that the neuritic plaques contain large amounts of a chemical called *beta amyloid protein*. A protein is simply a chain of amino acids, and as proteins go, beta amyloid is quite small, containing only about 40 amino acids. It has been shown to be toxic to nerve cells, and is thought to be central to the brain damage that occurs in Alzheimer's disease.

Beta amyloid protein is only a small fragment of a much larger chemical called *beta amyloid precursor protein*, which is present in all nerve cells and helps maintain connections between brain cells.

The gene for both these proteins resides on chromosome 21, and defects in this gene have been associated with familial Alzheimer's disease, in which plaques containing beta amyloid protein develop early, presumably because the genetic defect has caused the chemical to accumulate. In Down syndrome, an extra copy of this chromosome is present in every cell of the body. Those with Down should then produce higher than normal levels of beta amyloid protein, and indeed they have been found to develop many neuritic plaques containing this chemical in their late thirties and forties.

Though the role of beta amyloid protein in Alzheimer's is far from being completely understood, clearly this small chemical plays an important part in the mechanism of the disease.

involved in Alzheimer's because people with Down syndrome, who have an extra copy of the chromosome, develop the brain changes of Alzheimer's disease at an early age. Chromosome 21 carries the gene for beta amyloid precursor protein, the protein that, if altered, can produce beta amyloid, the chemical present in large amounts in the plaques and neurofibrillary tangles characteristic of Alzheimer brains.

- *Chromosome 19*: This chromosome is associated with late-onset Alzheimer's. Chromosome 19 also carries the gene for apolipoprotein E, which may be a risk factor.

- *Chromosome 14*: Mutations in this chromosome are associated with 70 percent of early-onset Alzheimer's.

Understanding genetics

Human characteristics are passed from generation to generation by *chromosomes*, rodlike structures found in every cell of the body. Every individual has a total of 46 chromosomes in 23 pairs, having received one chromosome of each pair from each parent.

Genes are the basic units that allow specific attributes or characteristics to be passed from one generation to the next. Each chromosome carries multiple genes, like beads on a string. *Alleles* are half-genes, and there are usually two for each attribute or characteristic, one from each parent. The combination of alleles received determines what characteristics will be expressed and which will be passed on to future generations. Some genes are *dominant* and others are *recessive*—that is, if the gene from one parent is dominant and the gene from the other is recessive, the person will show the dominant characteristic. But either gene can be passed to the next generation. Early-onset Alzheimer's is thought to be a genetic defect caused by the inheritance of an abnormal dominant gene.

- *Chromosome 1*: Mutations in this gene are also associated with early-onset Alzheimer's.

Alzheimer's Disease As Abnormal Metabolism

To function normally over a lifetime, the brain depends upon the production of proteins and other chemicals that work in harmony. Alzheimer's disease may in fact be an error of metabolism—that is, it may result from abnormal biological chemicals being produced, or normal biological chemicals being metabolized in ways that cause the buildup of waste products that damage neurons.

Genetic factors may be responsible, in that a gene may produce an abnormal or variant chemical that causes biological problems. This situation is well known in other diseases; gout is a good example.

It has been noted that a person with a genetic marker on chromosome 19 that codes for a specific type of apolipoprotein is much more prone to develop Alzheimer's disease. Apolipoproteins are molecules that are primarily responsible for transport-

Testing for the risk of Alzheimer's

It's possible to test for the presence of Apo E 4, but it's not a useful test for the disease. The presence of Apo E 4 cannot tell us whether someone will develop the disease; it merely gives us some idea of the likelihood.

In addition to this uncertainty, a person who is aware of an increased risk of Alzheimer's disease may suffer feelings of depression and helplessness and lose much enjoyment of life in worrying about a problem that has not yet appeared and may never appear.

ing fat within various organs, but are also important in healing inflammation within the brain. Abnormalities in apolipoproteins are associated with a markedly increased incidence of Alzheimer's disease. We inherit the two half-genes, or alleles, for apolipoprotein from our parents—one from our mother and the other from our father. There are three types of apolipoprotein allele—Apo E 4, Apo E 3 and Apo E 2—so various combinations are possible. People who inherit two copies of apolipoprotein 4 have almost eight times the normal risk of developing Alzheimer's. If only one copy of apolipoprotein 4 is inherited (from either parent), the disease occurs about three times more often than normal but starts later in life. Researchers have postulated that apolipoprotein 4 doesn't "work" biologically as well as the other apolipoproteins, and that this abnormal lipoprotein produces changes within the cell that initiate the cascade toward Alzheimer's. Apo E 2, on the other hand, seems to be protective— it decreases the risk of Alzheimer's.

Yet the situation isn't quite that simple. Some 15 to 20 percent of normal elderly people have two copies of the apolipoprotein 4 gene but no evidence of the disease. Furthermore, some elderly people who have Alzheimer's do not have any apolipoprotein 4 gene at all. Thus, the Apo E 4 gene is not always necessary for Alzheimer's.

Aluminum and Alzheimer's

Aluminum, in the form of aluminosilicate, is a common metal, making up 8 percent of the earth's crust. It is impossible to avoid, and is found in over three hundred different minerals. It's also found in cooking ware, cans, baking powder and foods such as cheese, tea and beer. Aluminum is easily absorbed through our skin, our gastrointestinal tract, our lungs and our nasal membranes. It has been shown to affect many different biological processes within the brain—as well as enzymes, DNA, intracellular structures and filaments, lipid membranes and neurotransmitters.

It has been suspected that aluminum may be associated with Alzheimer's disease for a number of reasons.

Aluminum May Be Toxic

Aluminum injected beneath the skin of rabbits causes degeneration of peripheral nerves, and when injected into the brains of rabbits or cats aluminum causes neuron damage and the formation of neurofibrillary tangles. (These tangles are not exactly the same as those found in Alzheimer's disease—they have straight filaments, not the paired helical filaments so typical of Alzheimer's.) High levels of aluminum have also caused dementia in people on kidney dialysis. These people showed intellectual deterioration, speech disturbance, muscle tremor and seizures, and at autopsy they were found to have increased aluminum in their brains (though not the characteristic tangles and plaques seen in Alzheimer's disease). Their dementia was discovered to be related to high concentrations of aluminum in the dialysis fluid, and some people were successfully treated by a therapy that removed the aluminum from their body. This *dialysis dementia*, as it was called, disappeared when dialysis fluids low in aluminum were used. Canadian miners exposed to aluminum dust (used as a preventative agent against silica-induced lung disease) developed dementia four and a half times more often than expected, suggesting that exposure to aluminum through the lungs was the cause. Workers exposed to excessive aluminum in a smelting plant suffered incoordination, poor memory, depression and impaired reasoning ability in direct proportion to the amount of aluminum they'd been exposed to. In short, there is no doubt that aluminum can be damaging to brain cells and brain function.

Alzheimer's Disease Brains Have a Higher Aluminum Content
The total body content of aluminum is in the range of only 30 to 50 mg, and the measurement of aluminum in the human brain is technically very difficult. This makes studies of measurements of aluminum difficult to compare. Earlier studies showed up to three times the normal level of aluminum in Alzheimer's disease brains. Newer studies in several laboratories have shown the aluminum content increased significantly in the areas of the brain affected by Alzheimer's (particularly the hippocampus), while other areas not involved in Alzheimer's have relatively little aluminum. More important, aluminum

Pots, pans and Alzheimer's

Though there may be increased levels of aluminum in the brains of people with Alzheimer's disease, the aluminum itself is probably not the primary initiating cause of the disease. Most likely, aluminum is picked up in excessive amounts in brains already damaged by Alzheimer's. There seems to be an association between aluminum levels in drinking water and Alzheimer's. But most experts agree that other exposure to aluminum, through aluminum pots and pans, or antacids and antiperspirants containing aluminum, does not cause Alzheimer's disease. As well, spouses and other family members of people with Alzheimer's do not have an increased incidence of the disease, suggesting that exposure to a common toxic element such as aluminum is probably not the only factor causing it.

appears to be increased in the neurofibrillary tangles and neuritic plaques characteristic of the disease. Increased aluminum is not seen in the brains of those suffering from other dementias.

Aluminum in Water

Aluminum can occur naturally in water, but it is relatively insoluble, so it settles to the bottom. Acidifying the water (which occurs with acid rain) increases the solubility of the aluminum and thus the amount absorbed by people who drink the water. As well, aluminum is added to water in the process of water purification, in the form of alum—a chemical that helps contaminants such as soil particles settle out. Many studies have shown that increased amounts of aluminum in drinking water are associated with an increased incidence of Alzheimer's disease. One study showed one and a half times more Alzheimer's in districts where the aluminum concentration in the water supply exceeded .11 mg per liter than in districts where the concentration was less than .01 mg per liter.

All in all, current scientific opinion suggests that aluminum may be important in Alzheimer's. It is probably not in itself the cause, but together with other trace elements it may possibly play a part, once the disease process has been set off by other factors that are not yet completely identified. If these other factors initiate a chain of events that allow aluminum to enter the brain in excessive amounts and to be metabolized in an abnormal way, there is no question that the aluminum could be toxic to brain cells and could contribute to neuron loss and inflammation.

At least one study showed mild to moderate improvement in the symptoms and signs of Alzheimer's disease when drugs were used to remove aluminum from the body. However, this is not a recognized medical treatment for Alzheimer's.

Brain Inflammation As a Cause of Alzheimer's

Inflammation within the brain plays a central role in Alzheimer's disease, but there is debate about whether this is the primary problem or whether it results from some other factor or disease process. The death of neurons, the formation of plaques and the accumulation of neurofibrillary tangles are all accompanied by some degree of inflammation within the brain, and this process is often referred to as a *cascade*, with one biochemical process following another. Many researchers believe that once the inflammation begins (from whatever cause), multiple biochemical abnormalities further damage the brain.

Researchers have noted that people with rheumatoid arthritis, who usually take large doses of anti-inflammatory drugs, have less than the expected incidence of Alzheimer's disease as they grow older, and when one identical twin takes anti-inflammatory drugs and the other doesn't, the one on the anti-inflammatory drugs is less likely to develop Alzheimer's. Even if the inflammation comes from some other cause, controlling it may very well lead to some hope for treatment of the disease.

Nerve-Growth Factors

Nerve-growth (neurotropic) factors are a group of naturally occurring proteins that regulate the survival, growth and function of neurons within the brain. These chemicals are decreased in the brains of people with Alzheimer's disease, and because these proteins protect brain cells and help them grow and survive, lack of them may be a cause of Alzheimer's. However, these nerve-growth factors are a diverse group of chemicals and are very difficult to measure. Their biology is such that they can't enter the brain from the blood and must be injected into the brain to have any effect. This obviously limits the possibility of treating Alzheimer's by supplying the factors, but some experimental treatments for the disease do use these compounds, extracted from animal brains, to counteract the inflammation seen in Alzheimer's.

The Free-Radical Theory

Free radicals are highly charged, unbalanced oxygen molecules that are constantly being released into the body by naturally occurring reactions. These molecules contain at least one unpaired (or "free") electron, and they "search" for another electron from some other chemical. They can cause damage because they can change the electron balance in essential cells of the body. Free radicals are part of the final common pathway of cell destruction and are linked to aging. They may play a role in neuron death following brain injury or damage, and thus may play a pivotal role in Alzheimer's disease. Researchers are working with anti-oxidants (such as vitamin E) to try to slow down the progression of Alzheimer's by decreasing the concentration of free radicals in the brain.

Other Possible Causes

Other theories about Alzheimer's disease have come into favor lately. Many are proposed to explain some of the defects seen in the disease. For example, disorders in calcium and iron metabolism have been demonstrated within the brains of people with Alzheimer's; zinc has been found to change certain proteins; in test-tube experiments these altered proteins damage brain cells and form plaquelike structures. Though these disorders of metabolism may be secondary to the inflammation of the disease, each of them has been proposed as a cause of the disease itself.

Stress is known to be associated with nerve damage in brain cells, through processes involving corticosteroids, and head injury or other neurological damage has also been proposed as an initial cause of the disorder because it can damage nerve cells and cause inflammation.

Some researchers believe that viral infections may be responsible for some or all of the inflammation of Alzheimer's.

NINE

Legal Issues

People with Alzheimer's spend the last years of their lives chronically ill, with mental and/or physical disability. Unless they make provisions for this eventuality, children, friends or strangers will be forced to make financial and health care decisions for them. Those who must make these decisions sometimes feel put upon because they may have no idea what the person would want. They could conceivably make choices the person never would have made. If others disagree it may lead to all-out war. For many it's a no-win situation. Whatever their decision, they will continually second-guess themselves, and live with doubt and guilt for the rest of their lives.

So it's in the interests of all—the person with Alzheimer's, and family, friends and health care professionals—to make the necessary arrangements ahead of time. With proper planning, those with the disease maintain some direction when they are no longer capable. The substitute decision-maker's job becomes easier and he or she can feel good about decisions implemented on the person's behalf.

The Will

The will is the basic document traditionally used to plan for the future. When someone is diagnosed with Alzheimer's it is important to make sure the person has a will. A will can be made by anyone over 18 who is considered to have testamentary capacity (competency to make a will). The person must understand the range of choices available and the implications of those choices. Witnesses to a will can be anyone 18 or older who understands the purpose of the document and does not benefit from the will. A will can be used for a variety of purposes: it can direct who should receive any particular property or possession; it can specifically request burial or funeral rites (be sure the executor is aware of this, or the will may not be read until it's too late); it can direct assets into a trust or to an attorney who will manage these assets for a child, disabled adult or someone else.

The will can be changed at any time, but a rule of thumb is that it should be written for a five-year span; then it can be completely rewritten, or a *codicil* can be added. A codicil is a legal document appended after the fact to save the inconvenience and expense of rewriting the whole document. There is no such thing as a simple will, and if a will is not drawn properly it can lead to lasting friction among family members. If there are a lot of small personal possessions to be distributed, the will can designate a trusted person to hand them out. The executor can then be told where to find a list telling this person who gets Grandpa's portrait, Aunt Molly's locket and so on. Because the list is not a legally binding document, it can be revised at any time, with no costs or formalities.

Draw up a will as early as possible after the diagnosis is made, with the aid of a lawyer. The lawyer ensures that the will truly represents someone's wishes, that all eventualities have been accounted for and that the will is an acceptable legal document. A will should be kept in a secure place where it can be easily obtained when needed. A secure place at home or in the lawyer's office is recommended; if it is kept in a safety deposit box at the bank there may be legal problems getting it after death, as boxes are sealed by banks in the event of death. This can delay the probate, the process that legally establishes the validity of the will.

The problem with the will is that it operates only when someone is dead. In the following sections are several legal ways in which people can work ahead to protect their interests *during* their lives, in the event of incapacitation. Properly used, they protect people's interests and save their families the emotional and psychological trauma of having to make decisions for the person with Alzheimer's.

Financial Planning

After retirement, most people cease to earn money. They aim to maintain both their security and their lifestyle by living off savings and pensions without diminishing their net worth. Most are concerned about distributing their assets fairly after death, and also want to ensure a smooth passage of resources, without too much shrinkage from government taxes. Proper financial planning aims to achieve all these goals. The need for such planning for someone with Alzheimer's is particularly urgent because Alzheimer's is an expensive disease and much of the care costs must be borne by those with the disease and their friends. Home care, nursing, transportation and institutional costs add up over the course of the disease. It's important to plan ahead to ensure that all assets are not used up.

As soon as the disease is diagnosed, get started. Organize finances. Find out about the person's bank account and safety deposit boxes. Know about his or her assets and liabilities, what his or her living expenses and debts are, what kind of pension plans he or she has. Plan for upcoming costs. If the person becomes incapable, it can be a nightmare trying to put the pieces together after the fact.

Checklist of original documents
Know where these documents are kept, for easy retrieval if necessary.

Personal	Yes	No	N/A
Birth certificate			
Driver's license			
Social insurance/social security no.			
Health insurance documents			
Marriage license(s)			
Military documents			
Divorce papers			
Will			
Spouse's will			
Power of attorney			

Financial	Yes	No	N/A
Savings account(s)			
Checking account(s)			
Safety deposit box keys			
Combination for safe			
Certificates of deposit/guaranteed investment certificates/savings bonds			
Insurance policies			
Property deeds			
Mortgages			
Bank loan(s)			
Credit card statements			
Income tax returns			
Retirement plans/pension			
Stock certificates			
Trust agreements			

Trusts

A trust is a means whereby one person (the *grantor*) transfers assets (*corpus*) into the name of another person or institution (the *trustee*). This may be appropriate for someone with Alzheimer's. The assets are handled as directed in the trust document. A trust can be created during the person's lifetime, or after his or her death, through the will. A *revocable* trust can be broken and the assets returned to the person's name; an *irrevocable* trust cannot be broken and the assets cannot be returned to the person's name or estate.

A trust can be simple or complex, depending on the needs. It is usually written by a lawyer to meet someone's specific needs and to ensure that it is legal. Trusts need to be signed by the grantor to be valid. There is no involvement with the courts unless the trust is challenged.

Trusts provide a way for older adults to have their assets professionally managed, without any need for guardianship (court intervention), in the event of incapacity. Trusts can preserve assets for the grantor's purposes in spite of mental incompetence later on, and can be used to shift income tax to a person in a lower tax bracket or to pass property on at death and avoid probate. They can continue through succeeding generations and are not subject to probate proceedings. The cost varies, depending on how complex the setup is. The trustee is entitled to a fee for managing the trust.

Power of Attorney

This is a legal document that allows the person executing the document (the *principal*) to hand over power to manage financial affairs to someone else (the *attorney*). The attorney doesn't have to be a lawyer; often it's a spouse, or a grown-up son or daughter. The contract is a very flexible arrangement. The attorney can receive sweeping powers or very specific powers. For example, someone can be given power of attorney to manage all financial affairs, or just to issue a check on a certain date in a certain place.

The power of attorney must be signed and witnessed. The laws in the jurisdiction where it's signed dictate how many witnesses must sign and who they can be. Some places require witnessing by one or two others, a notary public and/or registration with the government.

Since a regular power of attorney ceases if the principal becomes incapable, a *durable*, or continuing, power of attorney has been developed to extend the range of the power of attorney. This document includes a provision that it will remain valid even if the principal becomes incapacitated. Again, the attorney has the power to carry out only the business authorized in the document; he or she cannot do anything outside that range. Nonetheless, the contract can give the attorney sweeping powers over the principal's financial affairs, if that is what the principal wants. A durable power of attorney is recommended for people with Alzheimer's.

The principal should have complete confidence in anyone appointed as attorney. When granting power of attorney, it's important to understand:

• what assets are owned;
• what obligations are owed to dependants;
• that either a specific or a general power of attorney can be given;
• that a power of attorney can be revoked (canceled);
• that the attorney could misuse this power.

Legislation is now being passed across North America and Australia and in some European countries to broaden the range of issues covered by a power of attorney, so that not just finances and property but also personal care, health care and shelter are covered. This second type is called a "power of attorney for personal care." If there is any question about the capacity of the principal at the time the power of attorney is being granted, a letter from a doctor should accompany it. This letter should confirm that the person was capable and understood what he or she was doing. A power of attorney *cannot* be given once a person is incapable; it can only be given by someone who can understand the powers being given to the attorney.

Capacity and incapacity

The progressive erosion of memory and cognition caused by Alzheimer's diminishes the person's ability to think and reason. Capacity, or the ability to understand choices and appreciate the consequences of actions, is compromised. When is the person incapable of making choices and understanding decisions? That question is key. The challenge is to balance safety and freedom

Take, for example, Mrs. Green, an 84-year-old widow living alone. She had Alzheimer's and had been burning pots and pans. She had been taken home by the police twice because she got lost shopping. One of her daughters wanted to leave her at home, and accepted the risk of fire, accident or injury. Another daughter wanted to put her in a nursing home to keep her safe.

Mrs. Green insisted that she had no problems and that she would "rather die" than live in a nursing home. But she might be incapable of understanding her risks. She was still able to wash, dress and feed herself. If her daughter shopped and paid her bills, she might be able to cope. But she was not capable of performing more complex tasks, such as managing her money or traveling downtown to shop.

In practice, capacity usually involves some form of risk management. One daughter accepted risk; the other didn't. The mother's capacity was key: did Mrs. Green understand that she was at risk, and did she accept the risk? The goal was to preserve her freedom and minimize her risk. It's a complex balancing act at times.

A declaration of incapacity—sometimes involving formal testing and a physician's certification—is very serious. It removes someone's fundamental right to make choices. Incapacity must therefore be proved legally. "Bad choices" are not adequate reasons for declaring incapacity. Sometimes, by virtue of idiosyncrasy or eccentricity, capable people make choices that seem inappropriate to others.

The presence of Alzheimer's disease does not automatically render an individual incapable, particularly in the early stages. In the past, people with Alzheimer's were automatically considered incapable. While illnesses that affect intellectual functions may compromise capacity, this is not always the case. People must be assessed specifically for decision-making capacity, and not assumed to be incapable simply because they have Alzheimer's.

Guardianship

If someone with Alzheimer's becomes mentally incapable and has made no provisions, or has not planned for this development, a power of attorney cannot be granted. The person becomes a *ward* of the court and the court appoints a guardian to make decisions on his or her behalf. The incapable person then becomes a ward of the guardian. The guardian reports to the court and must submit documentation to support expenses claimed and decisions made. Guardianship is a much more expensive and complicated process than the durable power of attorney, and very few of us would want our families to go through it if it could be avoided.

Before someone is made a ward, he or she must be declared incapable in some or all capacities. (Someone might be capable of personal care, for example, but incapable in financial matters.) Once a legal judgment of incapacity has been made, according to the individual's circumstances, the ward may lose the right to make personal decisions: these may include the right to make contracts, to marry, to make health care decisions or to handle financial affairs.

The guardian is often a relative who applies to the court to become the ward's protector. The court reviews evidence of the ward's incompetence and considers whether guardianship is in his or her best interests. The person applying to become guardian argues why he or she is qualified and is the most suitable person to carry out that task. Guardianship may extend to include the ward's estate and finances, or personal decisions, or both. The guardian must obtain the court's approval to carry out certain transactions, such as the sale of the ward's home if the ward is admitted to an institution.

Advance Directives

Medical technology enables people to live longer than in the past, but often this extra time is spent with some form of chronic mental and/or physical disability. Unless this has been planned for, family and friends may have to make agonizing decisions.

Before people with Alzheimer's become incapable, they should make their wishes known. This will protect them, their family and their friends.

How can people get the health care *they* want if they become incapacitated? How can they let others know their wishes, and protect family and friends from the predicament of having to decide for them? Discussing these issues in advance can prevent conflict later. The drawback of informal discussions is that people may not recall them accurately. Years later, in a time of crisis, the family may have mixed opinions about what was said and meant. People can avoid this problem by clearly documenting their wishes in an *advance health care directive*.

What Is an Advance Health Care Directive?

An advance health care directive, or "living will," is a written statement that specifically expresses someone's wishes in regard to health care. It contains instructions about care in case the person is not able to make such decisions at a later date. It enables a person to state his or her wishes for medical treatment and personal care, and to grant someone else power of attorney in these areas.

As long as the person remains competent, able to consider and communicate health care choices, he or she will be able to make these decisions personally. A health care directive comes into effect only when someone is incompetent and unable to make his or her wishes known. There are two types—"instructional" and "proxy."

An *instructional directive* states which treatments are wanted or not wanted under given circumstances. These statements can be general or specific. The more specific the instructions, the easier they will be for family and doctors to follow. An instructional directive is not limited to the treatment of terminal or irreversible conditions. It can also apply to curable, reversible conditions. It can deal with health care decisions early in Alzheimer's, when the person has a good quality of life.

A *proxy directive* nominates a substitute (a *proxy*) to make decisions for health or personal care if someone becomes incompetent. This substitute has the ability to make these decisions in the same way that a substitute who has financial power of attorney can manage finances.

Are Health Care Directives Legal?

A health care directive is a legally binding document in most jurisdictions in North America. There may be a minimum age for the person substituting, or certain other restrictions. Depending on where you are, witnesses may be required. Some regions recognize proxy directives; others recognize both proxy and instructional directives.

Who Should Be Chosen As a Substitute?

The substitute must be someone who can be relied on, and someone who will likely be available to carry out the wishes. (An alternate may also be named, in case the substitute is not available.) Wishes for health and personal care should be discussed thoroughly with the person appointed. When this person understands what is wanted and can carry out all the wishes, written instructions should be left with him or her, as well. This person is then bound to follow the instructions, unless there is excellent reason to believe that circumstances would have caused the person granting the directive to change his or her mind.

"Let Me Decide"

The "Let Me Decide" directive was originally developed for people with Alzheimer's disease so they could plan ahead. This popular health care directive is now used worldwide to help adults of all ages plan their health and personal care. It consists of an introduction, a personal statement, a health care chart specifying wishes for treatment in various medical situations, some definitions of terms so that doctors can interpret those wishes correctly, and a name-and-address list. A copy of the directive is included at the end of this chapter. (For more copies see "Health Care Directive," in the Resources section at the end of this book.) The rest of this chapter explains how the form should be completed.

Introduction

This section explains why you are completing the directive, and advises others that the directive is not to be used while you are conscious and able to make decisions for yourself. It revokes any previous documents and establishes the directive as the current expression of your wishes. It also names a substitute decision-maker.

Personal Care Statement

This can address any area of health or personal care not covered elsewhere in the directive. Consider your statement carefully. The more specific it is, the easier it will be for others to follow.

Complete the introductory sentence, "I consider an irreversible condition to be any condition...," in your own words, to tell others what stage of Alzheimer's disease or level of disability you would consider unacceptable. Most people want different care depending on how intolerable their condition is. Specify as clearly as possible what *you* would consider intolerable.

This section can state your wishes regarding personal care, such as where you live, safety issues, clothing and hygiene. You can also make known your wishes about organ donation, post-mortem examination and cremation. If you're a Jehovah's Witness, be sure to include your instructions with regard to blood transfusions.

Health Care Chart
This documents your wishes for treatment in case of life-threatening illnesses, feeding problems or cardiac arrest. Different choices are made depending on whether your condition is acceptable, or irreversible or intolerable. For explanations of some of the terms used, see below. It's prudent to review these instructions with your doctor every year or so; space is provided for updated information. If you review your directive and make no changes, just write "no change" and sign and date it, with your doctor. If you change your wishes, you must tell your substitute(s), update all copies of the directive and have everybody sign them.

Definitions
This section explains a number of the terms used in the directive—for example: "irreversible/intolerable" (no possibility of a complete recovery, permanent disability, with poor quality of life, as in advanced Alzheimer's), or "acceptable" (without permanent disability, with good quality of life, as in early Alzheimer's).

Signatures
In this section, enter the names, addresses and phone numbers of your family doctor, substitute decision-maker(s) and witnesses. Include home and work numbers, along with any other numbers where these people can be reached in an emergency.

Life-Threatening Illnesses
Pneumonia is an example of an illness that may cause death. Although pneumonia may be fatal, most healthy people recover fully with treatment. Those with Alzheimer's and severe disability may wish to allow the pneumonia to run its course; they may not want antibiotics.

Donating your brain for Alzheimer's research

Many people want to help the research effort to untangle this puzzling disease. One way to help is to donate brain tissue. This tissue is carefully stored, then made available to researchers who study many different aspects, including new treatments and diagnostic procedures. Human brain banks are necessary because many serious neurological conditions affect only humans, and animal models are not available. Even normal brain tissue is vital, because it provides standard values for many chemicals and substances in the brain.

In Canada, contact the Brain Tissue Bank. In the U.S., samples are generally from patients who have taken part in research studies; to become involved, contact the Alzheimer's Association. (See Further Resources for details.)

People rarely die directly from chronic illnesses such as Alzheimer's. They are more likely to die from complications, such as pneumonia or blood clots to the lungs (pulmonary embolism). If a decision is made to treat life-threatening illness in someone with advanced Alzheimer's, more tests and investigations may be needed. This means blood tests, X-rays, injection or even surgery. All this can be uncomfortable or painful, and the treatment may only prolong the dying process. In these cases doctors often advise families to let the person die peacefully, to prevent further suffering. With an advance care directive, you yourself can state the level of care you would want in such a case.

Palliative care aims to keep people comfortable and to relieve pain. The goal is not cure, but comfort and relief from suffering. Tests and treatments are done not to prolong life but only to maintain comfort. People who have requested this level of care may have surgery, but only to improve their comfort or relieve pain. For example, if you broke a hip and had asked for palliative care, surgery could be done to pin the hip, if this was the most effective way to relieve the pain. But if you had bleeding in the stomach or intestine, you would not receive blood transfusions or drugs to stop the bleeding.

Limited care includes more treatment than "palliative" but less than "surgical." For example, if you developed pneumonia you could receive antibiotics, blood tests, intravenous fluids and X-rays. If you had bleeding in the intestine, you could receive blood transfusions and drugs to stop the bleeding. But you would not have emergency surgery to stop the bleeding, or medical tests calling for a general anesthetic. You would not be put on life-support machines. You would not go on a dialysis machine if your kidneys failed.

With *surgical care* you would receive blood tests, X-rays and surgery, and you would be put on a dialysis machine if you needed it. You would be put on a breathing machine during or after surgery if necessary. You would receive intravenous fluids and blood transfusions if you had life-threatening bleeding from, say, the bowel. A tube might be passed into the bowel (endoscopy) to find the cause of bleeding. If necessary, doctors would perform surgery to correct the bleeding.

At the *intensive care* level, doctors would consider any treatment that might keep you alive. That might include surgery, biopsies and life-support systems (dialysis machines, breathing machines), or even transplant surgery (including heart, kidney, liver or bone marrow transplants). If you were at home, you would be transferred to hospital; if you were in a small community hospital, you could be transferred to a larger hospital for more advanced diagnostic tests and treatments.

Feeding Problems

Many people in the later stages of Alzheimer's become unable to swallow, and choke on their food. If they can't swallow they must receive fluids or food artificially to stay alive. Someone must decide if and how they should be fed. There are four ways to feed them: basic, supplemental, intravenous and tube.

Basic feeding means spoon-feeding with a regular diet (fluids and solids). You would receive fluids if you were uncomfortable from thirst. (Dehydration can be very uncomfortable for conscious people.) People who can't swallow may receive *subcutaneous* (under the skin) or intravenous fluids, for comfort.

Supplemental feeding means basic feeding plus high-energy supplements or vitamins. Intravenous feeding is not used.

Intravenous feeding is for people whose intestines are not absorbing food; it means that fluids and food are given directly into the veins. This method works for a limited time only because the needles eventually damage the veins. When the veins in the arms can no longer be used, larger veins in the chest and neck are used, to get more food and fluids into the body.

Tube feeding uses *nasogastric* and/or *gastrostomy* tubes. Nasogastric tubes pass through the nose into the stomach, for people who can digest food but can't swallow. Most people tolerate them well, but some find the tubes uncomfortable and keep pulling them out. Gastrostomy tubes pass through the abdominal wall into the stomach, for people who can't tolerate a nasogastric tube, or who will need feeding for a long time. Gastrostomy tubes can be inserted without a general anesthetic. They are fairly painless and trouble-free.

Cardiac Arrest

Cardiopulmonary resuscitation, or CPR, is an emergency procedure that attempts to restore breathing and heartbeat when they have stopped. Decisions about CPR should be made in advance if possible. CPR includes pumping on the chest to keep the blood flowing through the heart, and mouth-to-mouth breathing or a breathing machine (mechanical ventilation). It may also include drugs and electric defibrillators (machines that shock the heart into action).

CPR was originally developed for people whose hearts had stopped from a heart attack, drowning or some other cause. If a healthy person's heart stops, there is a good chance that he or she can be kept alive until advanced medical care takes over. CPR can give this person many extra years of good-quality living.

In older adults with severe dementia, CPR is nearly always unsuccessful. The few people who do survive do not often live long. But hospital staff are required to do everything possible to save a person's life in an emergency. Unless clear instructions are given to the contrary, every patient is given CPR.

A "NO CPR" order says that no attempt at revival should be made when breathing or the heart has stopped. This order is becoming common as more and more people fear that medical technology will be used to prolong their lives artificially and leave them with a poor quality of life. Many would rather have a peaceful end when the time comes.

Personal Care Issues

In the late stages of Alzheimer's, we need others to assist with our personal care. We may require help with grooming, dressing, feeding, going to the toilet, shopping or choosing where

---

Organ donation

In the past twenty years, since drugs have been developed to prevent the body's rejection of transplanted tissue from other humans, organ donation has become widespread. Many of us know someone who is alive today only because he or she received a heart, lung, kidney, liver or bone marrow transplant. Some people who were blind can see again because of corneal transplants. Consider whether you'd like to donate your organs to others before making the personal statement in your health care directive.

to live. The substitute decision-maker nominated in the advance directive can make decisions about your personal care, but he or she needs to know what you would want. Do you feel strongly about wearing hospital clothes? Is hair care important to you, or frequent shaving? Should you be bathed or groomed against your will? Should you be allowed to eat what you like, or restricted to a healthy diet? What little luxuries really matter to you, and what can be sacrificed for the sake of convenience?

With Whom Should You Discuss Your Directive?
Discuss your directive with family, close friends and your doctor before you complete it, but make sure the final decision is yours, and not the result of pressure from others. It's a good idea to discuss these issues with your doctor because he or she may be called when you get sick. Your doctor should be able to answer any questions you have, and will be able to tell others your wishes if you want. You don't need a lawyer to complete this document, but you may want to let your lawyer know you have a health care directive when you're making out or updating your will. Leave a copy with your doctor and your substitute(s). If you wish, get photocopies and distribute them to your lawyer and family.

Let Me Decide
Health and Personal Care Directive

1. Introduction

In this Directive I am stating my wishes for my health and personal care should the time ever come when I am not able to communicate because of illness or injury. This Directive should never be used if I am able to decide for myself. It must never be substituted for my judgment if I can make these decisions.

If the time comes when I am unable to make these decisions, I would like this Directive to be followed and respected. Please do everything necessary to keep me comfortable and free of pain. Even though I may have indicated that I do not want certain treatments, I recognize that these may be necessary to keep me comfortable. I understand that my choices may be overridden if a treatment is necessary to maintain comfort.

I have thought about and discussed my decision with my family, friends and family doctor. In an emergency, please contact my power of attorney(s)/substitute decision-maker(s) or my family doctor listed below. If these people are not available, then please do as I have requested in this Directive.

I, _____, revoke any previous power of attorney for personal and health care made by me and APPOINT

_____

jointly and severally to act as my power of attorney (proxy, mandatory) and to do on my behalf anything that I can lawfully do by an attorney for personal care, including giving consent to treatment. If he/she/they is/are unable, unwilling or in the event of resignation, death, mental incapacity, refusal or court removal, then I appoint as alternate _____

_____ substitute(s), power of attorney(s) (proxies, mandatories) to act jointly and severally as my substitute(s) or attorney(s) for personal care.

[If you've named more than one substitute, (attorney, proxy, or mandatory) or more than one alternate and you want each of them to have the authority to act separately, leave the words "jointly or severally." If you want them to act together, not independently, delete "and severally" and leave "jointly." If you have named one person, delete "jointly and severally."]

Dated and signed this _____ day of _____ (year)_____

_____
Signature   Print Name   Health Card No.

2. Personal care

I would consider an irreversible condition to be any condition

_____

_____

_____

_____

_____

_____

_____

I would agree to the following procedures: (write YES or NO)

Blood Transfusion _____   Post Mortem _____

Organ Donation _____   Cremation _____

3. The Health Care Chart

If my condition is Acceptable			If my condition is Irreversible/Intolerable		
Life-Threatening Illness	Cardiac Arrest	Feeding	Life-Threatening Illness	Cardiac Arrest	Feeding
Palliative Limited Surgical Intensive	No CPR CPR	Basic Supplemental Intravenous Tube	Palliative Limited Surgical Intensive	No CPR CPR	Basic Supplemental Intravenous Tube

Date   Signature   Power of Attorney Signature(s)   Physician Signature

Update once a year, after an illness, or if there is any change in health

Date   Signature   Power of Attorney Signature(s)   Physician Signature

Date   Signature   Power of Attorney Signature(s)   Physician Signature

Date   Signature   Power of Attorney Signature(s)   Physician Signature

Date   Signature   Power of Attorney Signature(s)   Physician Signature

4. Definitions

Acceptable condition: Condition where I have an acceptable quality of life.

Irreversible/intolerable condition: Condition where I have intolerable or unacceptable disability (e.g. multiple sclerosis, stroke, severe head injury, Alzheimer's disease).

Feeding

Basic: Spoon-feed with regular diet. Give all fluids by mouth that can be tolerated, but make no attempt to feed by special diets, intravenous fluids or tubes.

Supplemental: Give supplements or special diets (e.g. high calorie, fat or protein supplements).

Intravenous: Give nutrients (water, salt, carbohydrate, protein and fat) by intravenous infusions.

Tubes: Use tube feeding. There are two main types.

Nasogastric tube: a soft plastic tube passed through the nose or mouth into the stomach.

Gastrostomy tube: a soft plastic tube passed directly into the stomach through the skin over the abdomen.

Cardiac Arrest (CPR)

No CPR: Make no attempt to resuscitate.

CPR: Use cardiac massage with mouth-to-mouth breathing; may also include intravenous lines, electric shocks to the heart (defibrillators), tubes in throat to lungs (endotracheal tubes).

Levels of Care

Palliative care
— keep me warm, dry, and pain free
— do not transfer to hospital unless absolutely necessary
— only give measures that enhance comfort or minimize pain (e.g. morphine for pain)
— intravenous line started only if it improves comfort (e.g. for dehydration)
— no X-rays, blood tests or antibiotics unless they are given to improve comfort

Limited care (includes Palliative)
— may or may not transfer to hospital
— intravenous therapy may be appropriate
— antibiotics should be used sparingly
— a trial of appropriate drugs may be used
— no invasive procedures (e.g. surgery)
— do not transfer to Intensive Care Unit

Surgical care (includes Limited)
— transfer to acute care hospital (where patient may be evaluated)
— emergency surgery if necessary
— do not admit to Intensive Care Unit
— do not ventilate except during and after surgery (i.e. tube down throat and connected to machine)

Intensive care (includes Surgical)
— transfer to acute care hospital without hesitation

— admit to Intensive Care Unit if necessary
— ventilate if necessary
— insert central line (i.e. main arteries for fluids when other veins collapse)
— provide surgery, biopsies, all life-support systems and transplant surgery
— do everything possible to maintain life

5. Signatures
Family Physician

Name: _____

Address: _____

Tel: (H) _____

Tel: (W)_____

Signature: _____

Power of Attorney(s)/ Substitute(s)/Proxy(s)

1. Name:_____

Address: _____

Tel. (H) _____

Tel: (W)_____

Mobile Tel:_____

2. Name:_____

Address: _____

Tel. (H) _____

Tel: (W)_____

Mobile Tel:_____

Witnesses
We are the witnesses to this power of attorney. We have signed this power of attorney in the presence of the person whose name appears above, and in the presence of each other, on the date shown above. Neither one of us is the attorney, a spouse or partner of the attorney, a child of the grantor or person whom the grantor has demonstrated a settled intention to treat as a child of the grantor, a person whose property is under guardianship or who has a guardian of the person, or less than eighteen years old. Neither one of us has any reason to believe that the grantor is inca-pable of giving a power of attorney for personal care or making deci-sions in respect of which instruc-tions are contained in this power of attorney.

1. Name:_____

Address: _____

Tel: (H) _____

Tel: (W)_____

Signature: _____

2. Name:_____

Address: _____

Tel: (H) _____

Tel: (W)_____

Signature: _____

TEN

Treatments for Alzheimer's Disease

Although there is no cure for Alzheimer's, drugs are now available not only to slow the disease's progress and improve memory but also to relieve depression, anxiety and anger. Used appropriately, these drugs can significantly improve the quality of life for both the sufferer and the caregiver. Used inappropriately, they can impair quality of life and make the condition worse.

When treating a person with Alzheimer's, it is important to set "goals of treatment." Since there is no cure, the goals of treatment are to improve function and quality of life. It is equally important to decide whether the main goal is to prolong life or to improve its quality.

Depression or anxiety should always be treated, because this can improve the person's function and quality of life. Treatment of a life-threatening illness is a more complicated issue. If pneumonia occurs in the early stages, treatment with antibiotics may be appropriate. But antibiotics may not be indicated in the late stages, when the person is bedridden and incontinent. Treatment in the late stages may just prolong the dying process. In severe Alzheimer's the goal of treatment is palliative care—preserving the person's dignity and trying to manage symptoms. We recognize that death is an inevitable consequence of this disease and we allow it to occur naturally.

The health care system has three goals. The first is to reduce disability by promoting health and prevention. The second is to screen ill people, judging which would benefit from treatment and which would not, to ensure that those who would benefit from treatment get it and those who would not avoid unnecessary, futile investigations and procedures. The third goal is to ensure that when people are severely disabled at the end of their lives, we allow them to die naturally, with a minimum of suffering. In the final stages of Alzheimer's, death can be a good outcome. After a long struggle with the disease, family and friends are often relieved when the person dies and his or her suffering is finally over.

One of the biggest growth areas in health care today is the quest to understand aging. Everyone wants to live longer and stay healthy and vital. There is great interest in treatments that slow aging and preserve health. Since Alzheimer's is common in old age, there is growing interest in finding drug treatments to prevent it, to stop its progression or to at least improve the memory and function of those who have it.

We can divide drug treatments into three broad categories:

- curative treatment
- preventive treatment
- symptomatic treatment

Curative Treatment

There is no cure for Alzheimer's at present. We don't know the cause, and we can't prevent the disease from progressing once it has started. Major research efforts continue, however, and scientists are making breakthroughs to identify the causes of Alzheimer's (see chapter 8).

Preventive Treatment

We can't prevent the disease yet, but as we learn more and more about it we are discovering treatments that may retard its progress once it starts. There are now four different treatments that seem to slow or delay memory loss in older adults.

Alzheimer's Vaccine

In December 2000, researchers published findings that when *transgenic* mice were injected with amyloid beta-peptides their cognition improved. (These mice have been bred and tested because they have a gene that causes them to get an Alzheimer's-like dementia. They are used as animal models to test different experimental treatments before the treatments are used in humans.) When the transgenic mice received these injections, there was a reduction in the amount of amyloid plaques in their brains.

Human trials then started in the United States and Europe, with several hundred patients, but had to be halted when some of the subjects developed inflammatory reactions in their brains.

Researchers continued to refine the vaccine, and discovered the part that stimulated antibodies and led to inflammation. The vaccine was modified and refined to prevent the antibody formation and inflammation. Research on the new, improved vaccine continues.

Estrogen

In women, the hormone estrogen has many powerful, different anti-aging properties. The use of estrogen as a supplement is controversial, however, because it has potentially harmful effects as well as benefits. There is some evidence that estrogen may prevent Alzheimer's in some women. Estrogen acts on the brain as a neurotropic factor, encouraging the growth and repair of neurons. It also increases the neurotransmitter acetylcholine and increases blood flow to the brain. In one study where 1,124 women aged 70 and over were followed for five years, 3 percent of those taking estrogen developed Alzheimer's each year, whereas 8 percent of those not taking the drug developed the disease. Long-term studies show that women who take estrogen age more slowly. But many women are afraid to take it because it may increase the risk of breast and uterine cancer and even stroke. Women with a previous history or strong family history of breast cancer should avoid estrogen. Consult your doctor.

Vitamin E

A recent study showed that vitamin E significantly slowed the progress of Alzheimer's. People with Alzheimer's were given either vitamin E, selegiline (a drug that affects brain chemicals), a combination of both or a placebo (an inactive compound) and were followed for about two years. The people taking vitamin E had slower memory decline than those who took selegiline, the combination or the placebo. The people in the study took 2,000 international units (IU) of vitamin E every day, in two doses of 1,000 IU each. This is much higher than the usual dose of vitamin E.

At present we do not know if vitamin E actually prevents Alzheimer's, or delays the age of onset, or simply slows down the progression. We need to see these findings replicated in other studies. We also don't know if a lower dose would have the same effect. The safety of larger doses of vitamin E, over the long term, is unknown.

Nonsteroidal Anti-inflammatory Analgesics (NSAIDs)

Recent studies suggest that inflammation may be present in the brains of those with Alzheimer's. Some researchers have gone as far as proposing that Alzheimer's disease is entirely caused by inflammation. Research suggests that anti-inflammatory drugs such as ibuprofen suppress inflammation and may actually prevent or slow the progress of Alzheimer's. Various different studies have shown that people who take these drugs regularly are less likely to develop Alzheimer's. Studies have shown that on average, brains age three years less in people who take these anti-inflammatory drugs compared with those who do not. We don't know which of these drugs works best or what dose should be taken. Some researchers feel that 80 mg daily of enteric-coated ASA (aspirin) may be enough. (ASA is also called "aspirin" in the U.S. In Canada "Aspirin" is a brand name.) At present we don't know if these anti-inflammatory drugs work together with estrogen to provide cumulative effects.

ASA (aspirin) can cause stomach bleeding. It can also increase the tendency to bleed. People who take it may notice that they bruise more easily. It should always be taken on a full stomach, because this reduces the chance of stomach ulcers and bleeding. The enteric-coated form is broken down more slowly and this too reduces the risk of stomach ulcers and bleeding. Consult your doctor before you start taking it regularly. Higher doses of ASA (aspirin), or drugs such as ibuprofen, can affect the kidneys, cause fluid retention and increase blood pressure. They should be taken only under the care of a physician.

Selegiline

This drug is used in the treatment of Parkinson's disease. For years it has been touted as an anti-aging drug. Although it does slow the progression of Alzheimer's, it is not generally used because it is less effective than vitamin E, is more expensive and has more side effects. Unfortunately, selegiline has no additive effects when combined with vitamin E. In fact, vitamin E alone is better than selegiline or the combination of vitamin E and selegiline. This suggests that these drugs may actually interfere with each other. This should sound a warning to those who take many different herbs and vitamins. Combinations may not be better than single drugs, and the combined effects may actually be harmful.

In the future, more and more people will likely take "anti-aging cocktails." These combinations are under study, but at present it seems that a regimen of vitamin E with enteric-coated ASA/aspirin, and estrogen for women, may be the most likely candidate to slow or perhaps even prevent Alzheimer's. Unfortunately, these combinations have not been studied enough that they can be recommended to the community generally. Consult your doctor before you start taking any of them.

Ginkgo biloba

Ginkgo biloba is an Asiatic tree with fan-shaped leaves and fleshy yellow seeds. The extract of *Ginkgo biloba*, referred to as EGb 761, is one of the most popular plant extracts used in Europe and Asia to improve memory. It has recently been approved in Germany for the treatment of Alzheimer's disease. How it works on the nervous system is not completely understood, but it seems to act as an anti-oxidant, similar to vitamins E and C. In one recent study, 309 people with Alzheimer's were given 120 mg of ginkgo daily for a year. Ginkgo was safe, and it appeared capable of stabilizing, even improving, cognitive performance in these people. This improvement was equivalent to six months' delay in the progression of the disease in one-third of the people. It is not known if higher doses will produce even better effects.

Symptomatic Treatment

Improving Memory
Memory loss is the earliest feature of Alzheimer's. All attempts at treating the disease have been aimed at improving memory. Since the nerves that manufacture the neurotransmitter acetylcholine are damaged in Alzheimer's, attempts have been made to increase the levels of this chemical in the brain in the hope that this will improve memory and decrease symptoms. Choline and lecithin are used to make acetylcholine, but studies using these substances for Alzheimer's have consistently failed to show any improvement.

How Acetylcholine Works
Acetylcholine is released into the tiny space between two nerves to allow a message to be passed between them. Neurologists now believe that the nerves that use this chemical are responsible for short-term memory. When the chemical is released, it is active for only milliseconds before it is broken down by an enzyme called *acetylcholine esterase*. Many different drugs are known to block acetylcholine esterase. These are called *anticholinesterases*.

Studies many years ago showed that a drug named physostigmine, an anticholinesterase, could block this enzyme and improve memory. The problem with physostigmine was that it lasted only a few hours and had to be given frequently. The search began for a drug that could be given by mouth, would last longer and would not have severe side effects.

Tacrine
One drug, tacrine, has been tested and shown to improve memory. But tacrine causes nausea and damages the liver, and people who take it have to have blood tests regularly to check

for liver damage. Many can't tolerate it. A proportion of those who tolerate the drug derive benefits, but many doctors feel that the effects are so small and the risk so high that they should not prescribe it. It is rarely used now except by people who have been on it for some time.

More recently, three new and better anticholinesterases have been tested and found to be better tolerated in people with Alzheimer's. None of them is a cure, but they may have significant beneficial effects for the person with Alzheimer's and the caregivers.

Donepezil

Donepezil improves the ability to perform activities of daily living such as dressing and washing. Overall, caregivers note an improvement in function. This drug slows the progression of Alzheimer's and improves memory, equivalent to about a one-year delay. It is well tolerated and is taken only once a day, usually at bedtime. The starting dose is 5 mg once a day. After four to six weeks, the dose is increased to 10 mg once a day. The main side effects are nausea, vomiting and diarrhea, which usually diminish after a few days. Some people experience a drop in their heart rate. This can be a problem. Only about 6 percent of the people who try the drug cannot tolerate it.

The drug is available only on prescription, and caregivers should learn how to take the person's pulse for the first few weeks after the drug is started. If the person becomes dizzy or the heart rate drops to below 50 beats per minute, stop the drug and consult with the physician.

Rivastigmine

Rivastigmine is a powerful acetylcholine esterase inhibitor that acts to increase the level of acetylcholine, and thus is similar in effect to tacrine and donepezil. It shows promise as a potential new treatment. The most common side effects are nausea, vomiting, headache, dizziness and low blood pressure. Started at 1.5 mg twice daily for one month, the dose is then increased to 3 mg twice a day. In clinical trials where this drug was used, the dose of the drug was increased very quickly (every two weeks) and there were a lot of side effects. Many of these side effects are avoided by increasing the dose very slowly. After 3 mg twice daily, the dose is increased by 1.5 mg increments every two months: for example, 3 mg in the morning and 4.5 mg in the evening for two months, and then 4.5 mg twice daily for two months; the next increase is to 4.5 mg in the morning and 6 mg in the evening, until the final increase to 6 mg twice daily. Someone who experiences side effects stops the drug until they pass, and then goes back to the lower dosage that was tolerated. If the drug has been discontinued for four or five days or more, the person has to go back to the starting dose again.

Galantamine
Galantamine is an anticholinesterase inhibitor. Galantamine improves memory, cognition, self-care and behavior. The most common side effects are nausea, vomiting, diarrhea, dizziness, agitation, headache, loss of appetite and weight loss.

The recommended starting dose, 4 mg twice daily (8 mg per day), is given for about four weeks. Then the dose is increased to 8 mg twice daily. In another four weeks, the dose can be increased to 12 mg twice daily.

Galantamine is taken with morning and evening meals. If the drug is interrupted for more than a few days, the person is restarted on the starting dose of 4 mg twice daily. The drug is available in 4, 8, and 12 mg tablets. This drug may work for people who have had strokes causing their memory loss.

A comparison of some common benzodiazepines

	Half-life	Advantages	Disadvantages
clonazepam	20 to 80 hours	can be given at low dose for chronic anxiety	stored in fat; builds up
diazepam	14 to 100 hours	—	stored in fat; builds up
lorazepam	10 to 20 hours	will not build up in case of overdose	—
oxazepam	5 to 20 hours	will not build up in case of overdose	—

Anxiety

Anxiety is common in Alzheimer's. It will probably affect everyone with the condition at some time during the course of the disease. The person feels apprehension, accompanied by bodily symptoms such as rapid breathing and rapid heartbeat. Being left alone is the commonest anxiety. Often anxiety can be dealt with by manipulating the person's environment or by counseling and reassurance, but there may be times when medication is needed.

Benzodiazepines

All benzodiazepines have the same actions and effect. The big difference between them is in the length of time they act in the body. "Half-life" is the name given to the time it takes to break down half the drug in the bloodstream. The longer the half-life, the longer the drug's effects.

Benzodiazepines are used for panic attacks, anxiety and agitation. Sometimes they cause problems. They may induce drowsiness, and in the elderly the half-life is often longer than stated. People who take them are more likely to have car crashes.

Withdrawal may occur weeks after the drug is stopped. Frequent use of short-acting benzodiazepines causes rebound anxiety, and in some people with Alzheimer's the drugs may increase aggressive behavior.

Buspirone
This drug is nonaddictive and does not cause withdrawal. It is effective but may take some weeks to start working.

Tricyclic Antidepressants
These are often used effectively in small doses to treat anxiety.

Beta Blockers
Beta blockers (usually propanolol) are generally used for high blood pressure and heart disease. However, they have been used successfully to treat anxiety.

Depression
Depression is common in people with Alzheimer's. Up to half the sufferers may become depressed. Depression reduces quality of life and makes memory loss even worse. The good news is that depression can be treated and improved with drugs.

Selective Serotonin Re-uptake Inhibitors (SSRIs)
Just as the neurotransmitter acetylcholine is involved in memory, the neurotransmitter *serotonin* is thought to be responsible for mood. Drugs that increase the levels of serotonin in the brain improve mood. The antidepressants now most widely used belong to the group that raise serotonin in the brain by blocking the re-uptake of the chemical once it is released.
- *Fluoxetine* is one of the most successful drugs in history. It is estimated that more than 11 million people around the world take fluoxetine. It is a treatment for depression and

is used by almost three million North Americans. Side effects include decreased appetite, nausea, agitation, reduced sexual desire and weight gain. It may be too stimulating for the elderly and cause sleep disturbance, and it may interact with other drugs.

- *Paroxetine* is similar to fluoxetine and may be better tolerated in older adults. It is more sedating than fluoxetine and decreases anxiety. It too may cause drug interactions, and should be taken with caution with other drugs.
- *Sertraline* is more sedating than paroxetine, and less likely to interact with other drugs. It is usually given at bedtime.
- *Citalopram* is widely used because it is well tolerated and safe.

Tricyclic Antidepressants

This class of drugs has been used successfully for decades to treat depression. The drugs increase the levels of neurotransmitters in the brain. Unfortunately, the elderly are prone to their side effects, which limits their usefulness; SSRIs are now the drugs of choice for depression in this age group. Examples of tricyclics are amitriptyline, doxepin, nortriptyline and desipramine. Common side effects include confusion, which can worsen the memory loss; dry mouth; sedation; constipation; low blood pressure; heartbeat irregularities. Some tricyclics, such as amitriptyline and doxepin, are not generally used in older people because of their side effects.

Monoamine Oxidase Inhibitors (MAOIs)

Monoamine oxidase is a chemical in the brain that breaks down neurotransmitters. Its level increases with aging and this may contribute to depression in later life. Drugs that block the action of this chemical are known to cure depression.

Moclobemide is the main drug in this class used for people in later life. It is an effective and safe antidepressant, given morning and noon. There are no food restrictions and few side effects.

The drug does not affect sexual function, as SSRIs do, so it is used in younger adults whose decreased sex drive is a problem.

Aggression

Anger may have a neurochemical basis related to serotonin levels, and may become a serious problem in Alzheimer's. Agitated and angry behavior may be due to:

- *environmental factors*: The person with Alzheimer's is less able to understand or adapt to changes in environment. For example, when admitted to hospital the person may become very disorientated and agitated because he or she cannot understand the reason for the change in surroundings.
- *the Alzheimer's itself*: Some people with Alzheimer's simply behave "badly" as a result of the way their brain has been affected by the condition. No amount of environmental manipulation will help this type of agitation.
- *delirium*: This medical condition is common in those with Alzheimer's. It is a sudden loss of brain function due to dehydration, infection, drug toxicity (for example, a tricyclic antidepressant) or other illness. Delirium usually causes inattentiveness and fluctuations in awareness. Agitation is frequently present. Delirium is often a medical emergency because of the underlying condition that has caused it. For this reason, a person with Alzheimer's who becomes agitated needs to be investigated to rule out or treat dehydration, infection, heart attack and other similar acute conditions. If manipulation of the environment is not successful, and provided an underlying medical condition is not present, drug therapy may be needed.

Neuroleptics

These major tranquilizers treat hallucinations and delusions and are used extensively with schizophrenics. In the past, neuroleptics were often used to treat aggressive behavior in

Alzheimer's. Chlorpromazine was the original neuroleptic discovered in the 1950s. It often decreases blood pressure excessively and causes heavy sedation. Other drugs in this class include haloperidol, thioridazine, trifluoperazine, flupentixol, thiothixene, loxapine and pimozide.

The most common side effect of neuroleptics is muscle rigidity, which can worsen mobility and function. This is called "drug-induced Parkinson's syndrome." The person develops a masklike face that lacks expression. The hand shakes and he or she does not lift the feet when walking but shuffles. The person may not swing the arms when walking. Other side effects may be uncontrollable tongue and mouth movements called "tardive dyskinesia."

Some of these drugs are sedating and can lower blood pressure, which could lead to falls. All have side effects and should be used cautiously, starting with the lowest possible dose and gradually increasing the dose to get the desired benefits without the negative effects.

Atypical Antipsychotics

These drugs have largely replaced the old antipsychotic or neuroleptic drugs in the management of aggression, agitation, delusions and hallucinations in people with dementia. They are as effective as the old antipsychotics but do not have many of their disabling side effects. The major advantage of atypical antipsychotics is that they are much less likely to cause tardive dyskinesia. Atypical antipsychotics are also less likely to cause rigidity, tremor and confusion. The following are three atypical antipsychotics currently used.

Olanzapine is a well-tolerated and effective treatment for aggression, delusions and hallucinations. The starting dose is 1.25 to 2.5 mg at suppertime, to a maximum of 5 mg per day.

For acute agitation and aggression the drug comes as a wafer that dissolves in the mouth.

Risperidone is given once or twice daily; the starting dose is .25 mg once or twice daily. The dose is then gradually increased up to 1 to 2 mg per day. Risperidone causes rigidity, nausea, low blood pressure and sedation. There is concern that this drug may increase the risk of stroke.

Quetiapine is a promising new treatment, but it has not been well studied in the elderly. The dose ranges from 25 to 100 mg per day, in single or divided doses. It is least likely to cause rigidity.

Hormone Inhibitors

Estrogen and progesterone have been used in aggressive men with Alzheimer's to inhibit the production of testosterone (the male sex hormone), thus reducing sexually inappropriate and/or violent behavior. They are occasionally combined with atypical antipsychotics for severe behavior problems.

Sedatives

Trazodone is widely used, at night, as a sedative for older adults with dementia; the dose is from 12.5 to 50 mg. Other sedatives such as temazepam can also be tried. Many people with sleep problems try melatonin; some do well, while others seem to have no response or can't tolerate it. Melatonin is not legal in Canada, and is therefore not inspected; supplies bought illegally may not be safe. The drug is legal in the U.S.

Anticonvulsants

Antiseizure drugs such as carbamazepine have been helpful for dealing with aggression. Blood levels of these drugs can be monitored by a physician.

Non-drug Treatment

The importance of non-drug treatments cannot be over-stated. Caregivers need simple techniques to manage the range of difficult behaviors exhibited by people with Alzheimer's. A variety of non-drug therapies such as acupuncture, acupressure, massage, healing touch and therapeutic touch are widely used. Many such therapies have not yet been studied enough to warrant general recommendation, and some are based on theories that do not agree with established scientific principles.

Still, many caregivers say that both they and the people they care for have benefited from these techniques, and you may find some of them helpful. If the methods help both of you to relax and deal with the difficult aspects of your lives, you may not care too much whether the theoretical principles are valid. Just remember that some of the unproven therapies are expensive and aggressively marketed; if you aren't sure something is worthwhile, consult your doctor.

Healing by Touch

Healing by touch is as old as the hills. It has origins in every culture. The Scriptures mention the laying on of hands, and it is found in Asian, Polynesian, Indian, Egyptian, Native American and Celtic cultures. In modern times a wide variety of touch therapies are in use, including Japanese reiki and Chinese gigong. The theory behind healing touch is that each living organism has energy fields, and these fields are connected. Illness is thought to occur when an imbalance, shift or change in an energy field takes place. The goal of the healer is to use his or her own energy, along with the client's, to restore the balance or repattern the energy field so that the body can heal itself. This technique is noninvasive, does not use technology and has no harmful side effects.

Going to the dogs

When someone with Alzheimer's is withdrawn and unwilling to talk, it may be time to bring in the experts in nonverbal communication: dogs. Volunteer organizations arrange for gentle, disciplined dogs (and their owners) to have private visits with patients in hospitals and nursing homes. The dogs' affectionate, non-judgmental presence often stirs fond memories and may encourage the person to respond—first to the dog, and perhaps later to a therapist. Someone living at home may also react well to visits from a calm, manageable dog. Be patient—it may take weeks or months before the person really responds to the animal. As long as the encounter seems to give pleasure, it's worth pursuing.

Similar principles lie behind many different therapeutic techniques such as acupuncture, acupressure, reflexology, massage therapy, shiatsu and therapeutic touch.

Other Useful Approaches

Le Shan is different from the foregoing therapies in as much as it is based not on energy theory but on the healer's attaining an enhanced state of consciousness in order for a "flow process reality" to occur. Practitioners of Le Shan believe that everyone has a natural ability to heal, which can be accessed through this technique. In shamanism, the shaman heals by intuition and imaging using an enhanced state of knowledge that is obtained by stimulants, chanting, meditation, dancing and swaying.

Music therapy, aromatherapy and other routes to relaxation provide powerful ways to let go of frustration. They may help someone feel whole again. These techniques are being used more and more for people with Alzheimer's.

Summing Up

The challenge of helping a person with Alzheimer's disease remains to understand the person's problems, to continue to communicate and to keep the person engaged in the world.

Try to give love, respect and quality of life, but keep yourself healthy and vital, and find meaning in the experience. Drugs may help you manage the person's anxiety, depression and aggression, but they supplement other strategies and are never a solution alone. The solution to this disease is not found in a pill bottle—it's more complex than that! And remember, Alzheimer's is a journey that offers valuable opportunities and lessons, if we are ready to accept and learn them.

Some Drugs for Symptomatic Treatment of Alzheimer's

Generic name	Some brand names	Action
Aggression		
Olanzapine	Zyprexa	atypical antipsychotics
Olanzapine (sublingual)	Zydis	
Quetiapine	Seroquel	
Risperidone	Risperdal	
Chlorpromazine	Largactil	neuroleptics
Flupentixol	Fluanxol	
Haloperidol	Haldol	
Loxapine	Loxapac	
Pimozide	Orap	
Thioridazine	Mellaril	
Thiothixene	Navane	
Trifluoperazine	Stelazine	
Cyproterone	Androcur	hormone inhibitor
Estrogen	Premarin	
Temazepam	Restoril	sedative
Carbamazepine	Tegretol	anticonvulsant
Anxiety		
Buspirone	BuSpar	neuroleotic
Clonazepam	Klonopin*, Rivotril†	sedatives
Diazepam	Valium	
Lorazepam	Ativan	
Oxazepam	Serax	
Trazodone	Desyrel	
Depression		
Citalopram	Celexa	selective serotonin re-uptake inhibitors (SSRIs)
Fluoxetine	Prozac	
Fluvoxamine	Luvox	
Paroxetine	Paxil	
Sertraline	Zoloft	
Amitriptyline	Elavil	tricyclic antidepressants
Desipramine	Norpramin	
Doxepin	Sinequan	
Nortriptyline	Aventyl, Pamelor*	
Moclobemide	Manerix	monoamine oxidase inhibitor (MAOI)
Poor Memory		
Donepezil	Aricept	anticholinesterases
Galantamine	Reminyl	
Rivastigmine	Exelon	
Tacrine	Cognex	

*Available in U.S. only   †Available in Canada only

Glossary

Acetylcholine: a neurotransmitter, markedly decreased in Alzheimer's disease.

Agnosia: loss of the ability to identify everyday objects and their uses.

Amyloid precursor protein: a protein in normal brain cells that chemically metabolizes in Alzheimer's disease to produce beta amyloid.

Anomia: inability to find exactly the right word, or to name familiar objects.

Apolipoprotein: brain chemicals responsible for transporting fat and healing inflammation within the brain; important in the mechanism of brain damage in Alzheimer's.

Apraxia: inability to carry out purposeful movements and actions despite intact motor and sensory systems; inability to use an everyday object properly despite being able to identify it.

Association areas: anatomical and functional areas where information from various areas of the brain is integrated.

Atherosclerosis: "hardening of the arteries," narrowing of these vessels by deposits of fatty materials on their inner surfaces; the cause of most strokes.

Atrophy: wasting away of tissues.

Axon: a projection from a neuron whose function is to transmit information to other neurons.

Benign forgetfulness: a common and innocent pattern of memory loss for inconsequential events and details, commonly seen in the aged.

Beta amyloid: an abnormal protein that accumulates in the brains of Alzheimer's patients.

Capgras syndrome: a delusion common in Alzheimer's; the patient believes a spouse has been replaced by an identical impostor.

CT scan: computerized axial tomography: an X-ray technique commonly used in Alzheimer's, producing an image of the brain by computerized assembly of X-ray images.

Catastrophic reaction: a sudden, often violent outburst of anger and frustration resulting from a seemingly trivial provocation.

Circumlocution: literally "talking around"; a coping mechanism in early Alzheimer's disease, to paraphrase a correct word that cannot be recalled.

Cortex: the outer layer of the human brain, containing the cell bodies of the neurons.

Creutzfeldt-Jakob disease: a rare but severe and rapidly progressive form of dementia, felt to be due to an infectious particle as yet unidentified.

Dementia: a loss of such mental functions as memory, insight, judgment and reasoning ability; failure of the higher functions of the brain.

Dementia pugilistica: a dementia common in boxers, caused by repetitive blows to the head.

Dendrite: one of many tiny finger-like projections from a neuron, whose function is to receive information from other neurons.

Echolalia: the involuntary repetition of a word or phrase.

Encoding: the initial process of forming a memory, by recognizing that something is significant enough to notice and focusing on learning it.

Facilitation: reinforcing a memory by frequently recalling and reusing the information.

Free radical: highly charged, unstable oxygen molecule, thought to be important in causing inflammation and tissue damage and thus aging.

Frontal lobe: the front division of the cortex of the human brain, responsible for planning, insight and personality.

Frontal lobe dementia: a dementia characterized by progressive deterioration of personality and breakdown in social behavior.

Hippocampus: an area near the temporal lobe of the brain, responsible for short-term memory, and damaged early in Alzheimer's.

Hydrocephalus: a disease of the brain resulting from accumulation of cerebrospinal fluid, the liquid that bathes the brain and spinal cord.

Immediate memory: the ability to recall information that has just been presented.

Infarction: death of tissue as a result of inadequate blood supply.

Limbic system (limbic lobe): that part of the brain concerned with emotional control.

Long-term memory: the ability to recall, at will and over an extended period of time, information stored in the brain.

Melatonin: a hormone secreted by the brain, responsible for preparing the body for sleep.

MRI: magnetic resonance imaging; a highly sensitive technique producing an image of the brain using a magnetic field.

Neuritic plaque: characteristic accumulation of amyloid and cellular debris between brain cells in Alzheimer's.

Neurofibrillary tangles: groups of threadlike fibers found in brain cells damaged by Alzheimer's.

Neuroglia: brain tissue that supports and nourishes the neurons.

Neuron: nerve cell of the brain.

Neurotransmitters: brain chemicals found between neurons, which transmit information from one brain cell to another.

Occipital lobe: the part of the cerebral cortex at the back of the brain, responsible for vision.

Parietal lobe: the part of the cerebral cortex at the top and back of the brain, responsible for integration of the senses and the ability to calculate.

PET scan: positron emission tomography—a technique producing an image of the functioning brain by using radioactive tracers which are absorbed by working brain cells.

Pick's disease: a dementia involving mainly the frontal and temporal lobes, characterized by emotional instability and loss of inhibition.

Short-term memory: the ability to recall, over a short period of time, information held in the brain for rapid retrieval.

Stroke: sudden brain damage caused by blockage of the brain's blood supply or bursting of a blood vessel in the brain.

Sundowning: a pattern of increased confusion and agitation seen at night in Alzheimer's.

Synapse: the microscopic space between neurons, where impulses are transmitted from one brain cell to another.

Temporal lobe: the part of the cerebral cortex located on the side of the brain, responsible for speech and memory.

Further Resources

Organizations

U.S.

Alzheimer's Association
919 North Michigan Avenue
Suite 1100
Chicago, IL 60611-1676
(312) 335-8700
Fax: (312) 335-1110
Toll-free: 1-800-272-3900
www.alz.org

Canada

Alzheimer Society of
Canada
20 Eglinton Avenue W.
Suite 1200
Toronto, ON M4R 1K8
(416) 488-8772
Fax: (416) 488-3778
Toll-free: 1-800-616-8816
www.alzheimer.ca

Canadian Brain Tissue Bank
University of Toronto
UHN-Toronto Western
Hospital
399 Bathurst Street
Fell Wing 5-222A&B
Toronto, ON M5T 2S8
(416) 978-5490
cbtb@uhn.on.ca

Douglas Hospital Research
Centre Brain Bank
6875 LaSalle Boulevard
Verdun, PQ H4H 1R3
(514) 761-6131
brainbank@douglas.mcgill.ca

Maritime Brain Tissue Bank
5955 Jubilee Road
Room 1308
Halifax, NS B3H 2E1
(902) 473-2490

Books

Buckingham, R. *When Living Alone Means Living at Risk.* New York: Prometheus, 1994.

DeBaggio, Thomas. *Losing My Mind: An Intimate Look at Life with Alzheimer's.* New York: Free Press, 2002.

Honel, Rosalie Walsh. *Journey with Grandpa—Our Family's Struggle with Alzheimer's Disease.* Baltimore: Johns Hopkins, 1988.

Hamdy, R.C., J.M. Turnbull, W. Clark and M. Lancaster. *Alzheimer's Disease: A Handbook for Caregivers.* St. Louis, Missouri: Mosby, 1994.

Hodgson, Harriet. *Alzheimer's—Finding the Words.* Minneapolis: Chronimed, 1995.

Mace, N., and P. Rabins. *The Thirty-Six-Hour Day.* Baltimore: Johns Hopkins, 1981.

McGowin, Diana Friel. *Living in the Labyrinth.* New York: Delacorte, 1993.

Molloy, D.W. *Let Me Decide.* Hamilton, Ontario: New Grange, 1998.

Molloy, D.W. *What Are We Going to Do Now?* Toronto: Key Porter, 1996. Published in the U.S. as *Helping Your Parents in Their Senior Years.* Buffalo: Firefly, 1997.

Rhodes, Ann. *Help and Advice for Caregivers.* Toronto: HarperCollins, 1997.

Temes, Roberta. *Living with an Empty Chair: A Guide through Grief.* New York: Irvington, 1984.

Wilkinson, Beth. *Coping When a Grandparent Has Alzheimer's Disease.* New York: Rosen, 1992.

Health Care Directive

Copies are available from Let Me Decide, 440 Orkney Road, RR #1, Troy, Ontario, Canada, L0R 2B0. Telephone (905) 628-0354; Fax (905) 628-4901; www.netcom.ca/~idecide.

Videos

(You may be able to get these from your local Alzheimer's society.)

Dancing Inside. Auguste Productions Inc. Hoechst Marion Roussel.

Grace. University of Maryland at Baltimore.

Just for the Summer. McIntyre Media Limited, Rexdale, Ontario.

Prescription for Caregivers—Take Care of Yourself. Terra Nova Films Inc. Toronto, Ontario.

Index

Page numbers in italic indicate a figure, table or boxed text. For drug brands please see table of drug names on page 205.